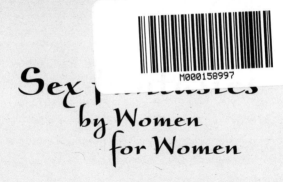

Sex Fantasies
by Women
for Women

Sex fantasies
by Women
for Women

edited by Lisa Sussman

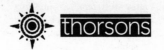
thorsons

Thorsons
An Imprint of HarperCollins*Publishers*
77–85 Fulham Palace Road,
Hammersmith, London W6 8JB

The website address is:
www.thorsonselement.com

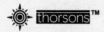

and *Thorsons* are trademarks of
HarperCollins*Publishers* Ltd

First published as *In Your Wildest Dreams* by Thorsons
in association with Cosmopolitan magazine 2001
This edition published by Thorsons 2003

8

© The National Magazine Company Ltd 2001

Lisa Sussman asserts the moral right to
be identified as the author of this work

A catalogue record of this book
is available from the British Library

ISBN-13   978-0-00-714743-4
ISBN-10   0-00-714743-0

Printed and bound in Great Britain by
Clays Ltd, St Ives plc

contents

Acknowledgements vii
Introduction ix

CHAPTER 1
Fantasy Foreplay 1

CHAPTER 2
Brief Encounters 28

CHAPTER 3
Sex with Another Woman 53

CHAPTER 4
Forced Fantasies 77

CHAPTER 5
Watching and Being Watched 102

CHAPTER 6
A Walk on the Wild Side 127

CHAPTER 7
Forbidden Thrills 154

CHAPTER 8
The Male Mind 176

CHAPTER 9
Sharing Your Fantasies 203

CHAPTER 10
Living Them Out 226

Acknowledgements

This book could not have been written without the help of my wonderful editor, Natalia Link, who used her red pen sparingly, and the open-minded insight of Samantha Grant and Wanda Whiteley.

Various professionals and organizations ensured that my information was accurate and up-to-date. I gratefully thank The Society for the Scientific Study of Sex, The Kinsey Institute and The Sexuality Information Education Counsel of the United States for liberal access to their libraries.

Also, eternal gratitude to the Sexual Health Information Center (*www.sexhealth.org*), *www.erotica.com*, and the newsgroup alt.sex for allowing me to post requests for contributions on their sites.

Thanks too to the campuses of Columbia University and New York University in New York City, Brown University in Rhode Island and Boston University in Massachusetts who allowed my requests for fantasies to remain unvandalized on their various message boards.

A note to the Hot Babes (you know who you are) – because of your efforts, that first e-mail calling for help eventually went around the world.

And to all the women and friends who revealed their secret desires – thanks. I hope all readers of this book will be as enriched by their generous sharing as I have been.

introduction

Newsflash: EVERYONE fantasizes – your lover, your boss, even your grandmother. In fact, there's a chance that they're doing it right now. Studies have discovered that 95 per cent of us have sexual fantasies daily. And for good reason – there are, after all, only so many ways we can touch or be touched lovingly in lovemaking. But since fantasy has no limits, our mental erotic wanderings become a creative expression of our sensuality.

It was once believed that people who fantasized didn't get enough sex or were lacking as lovers. As little as 30 years ago, women weren't even thought to do something so base as fantasize. It's now known that not only do real women let their erotic imaginations wander, but also that it's the people who are having lots of sex – and good sex at that – who are fantasizing the most. So dream on.

I sent out requests to real women and men to reveal their sexiest imaginings. Hundreds responded in uninhibited, explicit detail – by letter, e-mail and in person. To ensure full disclosure, respondents were told the inclusion of their names and any personal details was optional.

So what kind of fantasies does it turn out we're having? You name it. A fantasy is nothing more than a capricious wish, a picture or story you carry in your mind. It can be relaxing, exciting or arousing. It may be triggered by a thought, a scent, a glimpse of an erotic picture, the touch of a stranger's hand – anything that stirs your imagination. Some are but fleeting images – a breast, a thigh, a penis, a naked foot. Others are extremely intricate and detailed scripts. Women's fantasies lean towards being sultry, sensuous, steamy, and slow – an involved storyline that emphasizes caressing, conversation, and caring. By contrast, the typical male fantasy is a lot like a mental pornographic film. Forget foreplay and flirting. Forget the relationship, period. It's extremely visual and the point is instant physical gratification.

In the course of researching this book, I heard women's fantasies that involved a hundred kisses from head to toe, masturbating in front of a roomful of guys, being tenderly caressed by the Spice Girls, being lovingly licked by a golden retriever, seducing the young son of a neighbour, and being raped by a gang of teenagers. And I heard men fantasize about watching their partner have sex with someone else, overpowering a schoolgirl, being seduced by two or more women and having an anonymous quickie on a train. While many overlap, I divided the fantasies into what is generally acknowledged by experts as the top fantasy 'themes', each with a brief explanation exploring the underlying psychological urges that may have created this erotic longing.

But the real point is that fantasies come in many flavours and varieties. There is nothing forbidden or abnormal in what you do, say or think in the privacy of your mental passions –

and no limit to the pleasures you can explore and enjoy when you give free reign to your deepest desires. You may fantasize about having sex with the dustman, the dustman's wife or even the dustman's dog and still be considered an upright citizen with perfectly healthy sexual cravings. Whatever tips you off, it's fine to fantasize about. Your fantasies should only be a concern when they become compulsive or exclusive to the point of dominating your life.

In fact, fantasies are an essential part of our sexual repertoire. They make us more confident and satisfied lovers by liberating us and allowing us to be better than we really are; that is, more experienced, more confident, more risky, more desirable. They provide us with a safe means of exploring our wild side without fear of hurting our lovers or ourselves. You can safely satisfy your curiosity to know more about what it's like to be forced to have sex, to have sex with a friend or a relative, to make love in a public place or with another woman – even if these are things you would never consider doing in reality.

Consider the possibilities. You can look any way you want: beautiful, exotic, tall, blonde, dark-haired, busty, thin – anything at all. Your fantasy partner can be a celebrity, the guy who works down the hall, or your best friend's lover. You have complete control. You can write and direct the scene to play out any way you desire.

Your sexual flights of fancy are also a strong mental aphrodisiac. Masturbation and fantasies often go hand in hand (so to speak). But 80 per cent of people also use fantasies as a sexual accessory, to heighten the mood and help them focus when making love. Studies have also found that fantasizing prepares your body for a more powerful orgasm. The erotic images your mind conjures up increase circulation and muscle tension, allowing for more physical sensation and a greater feeling of release when you climax.

Simply put, sexual fantasies generate erotic energy and that energy is a wonderful gift you can give yourself. Use this book to read by yourself as a sexy pleasure just for you or to read aloud with the man you love to spur your sex life to new heights. Either way, enjoy!

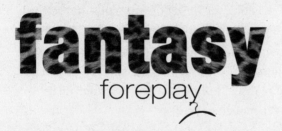

fantasy foreplay

Introduction

Each morning as you walk past his desk at work, the smell of his aftershave triggers an endless stream of fantasies. Whether you ever go out with him or not isn't the point. Many women stoke their desire by fantasizing about people in their everyday lives, especially if the person is attractive. It's a way of keeping life interesting and/or overcoming the sexual limits of a real-life relationship.

A twist on the crush fantasy is imagining that you're in a love scene with a celebrity, such as a movie star or singer. Sexual charisma is part and parcel of being famous. So fantasizing about a night of wild passion with George Clooney is just an extension of this star quality. Maybe some day you will meet George and you'll get to make mad passionate love with him. In the meantime, if you fantasize about George, then at least you can have him whenever you want.

Of course, no one really knows what sort of lover your fantasy really is, but who cares? The key issue here is desire. Because it's a fantasy of your making, there's no chance of you

1

being rejected – whether the object of your fancy is a celebrity or just someone you have desired for a long time. This is why this particular fantasy is often an ego-stoker for women when they're feeling unsure of their seductiveness. He might not give you a glance in real life, but in your fantasy, your imaginary lover just can't get enough of you!

He's baaaaack. Fantasizing about getting off with an ex-boyfriend takes this concept one step further. Here, you have a real and sometimes unhappily-remembered history with your dream lover. Fantasizing about them can be a way of working through your rejection or simply remembering explosive sex without dealing with the pain of relationship. It's the old 'could-have, would-have, should-have' thing. On the other hand, if sex with your ex was great, you may want to re-live it, perhaps using those memories to bolster your confidence in yourself as a lover.

Janine, 31, solicitor

In reality, my husband can't keep his hands off me. But my body is a real blocker to me seeing myself as sexual. I cannot imagine that a man would ever respond sexually to this body, these thighs. During sex, I have to imagine myself as younger, more agile, and with a very different physique in order to become more aroused.

Other fantasies I have are my husband sneaking up on me

while I'm sleeping and him giving me an oral surprise of a hundred kisses from head to toe.

Miranda, 29, estate agent

It's late and there's only me and my married boss left in the office. He looks over and gives me a lingering stare, so I stride over to him, hitch up my pinstripe skirt (we have to dress very formally at work) to reveal stockings and suspenders. We then have rampant sex on his desk.

Linda, 27, marketing consultant

My ideal man is handsome, powerful, intelligent, tender, loving. My current lover doesn't exactly match the profile, but who says I have to give up the fantasy? When I'm having sex with Ron, I just mentally project my fantasy like a romance movie. The fantasy excites me even more, which excites Ron, pushing our lovemaking to the heights of eroticism. Sometimes I feel guilty using fantasy while I'm making love with my lover, but what's the harm?

Sandra, 29, restaurateur

The alarm rings. Time to drag the bones out of bed and hustle to work, but the only thing rising is my lover – well, part of him anyway. He always wakes up at the ready. I'm flattered, amused, aroused. But ... work. He reaches for me, pulls me against his warm body, flicks his tongue over my nipples, strokes my clitoris. The clock is ticking. Forget long, lingering foreplay; the boss wouldn't understand. No time for other juicy, delicious lickings. Afterplay in the shower is steamy, but forget breakfast. I have my sweets in bed.

Denise, 24, receptionist

It's a very cold December day. I am wearing a heavy turtleneck sweater, leggings, and underneath it all, my sexiest teddy. He had called to meet with me – he being a local policeman. A very married policeman. I'd met him at work and we'd started out as friends, but soon moved on to lovers. 'Where?' I asked. It had to be somewhere on his beat but far enough from the centre of town that no one would catch us. We agreed on a park at the north end of town. When I arrive, we fall into each other's arms, kissing and undressing each other in a frenzy. It's probably minus 5°C outside, but we make wild, passionate love right there on the ground.

Daisy, 25, network analyst

My lover and I set the assignation. The hotel room is reserved. We tell our secretaries we'll be out for a lunch meeting. Like kids who successfully put one over on strait-laced grown-ups, we meet at the hotel.

We've agreed that the first to arrive orders room service for two. After all, lunchtime sex takes some planning and organization. Once we're both in the room, we waste no time with small talk. We're in the sack and in orgasmic ecstasy. No beepers, office phones, computerized calendars, machines – just our bodies, breath, odours.

After a non-stop morning at the office, staring into a computer monitor and dealing with aggravating trivia, this is pure animal sensuality. Nothing like a little sex fantasy for a mini-vacation in the midst of the workday.

Caroline, 34, manager

I am a divorced woman living quietly at home with my five-year-old daughter. Until recently, there hasn't been a man in my life. But since I met Matthew a year ago, I've become sexually active in ways I couldn't have imagined. One of our sexual escapades was so exciting that it has become a favourite fantasy I replay when I'm home alone.

In this fantasy, I remember every little detail about the first car trip we ever took together. It was a long drive. When Matthew was behind the wheel, I started feeding him a juicy hamburger and fries. He would lick and suck on my fingers as he took the food into his mouth. He kept his hands on the wheel and his eyes on the road, but pretty soon my hands were roaming all over his body. Just after dusk, we pulled over at a rest stop and wound up making love butt-naked in a grassy field.

Now, if anyone from work ever found out about that wild night, they'd say, 'Who would have thought it?' That's part of the fun – knowing how out of character this was for me and just how much I enjoyed it.

Laura

It's early morning and the sun is attempting to creep into the room from behind the closed blinds. It's Saturday, and I thought you could use a little extra sleep, so I've been quietly moving about, careful not to disturb your slumber. From time to time you shift your body under the warm comforter and finally end up on your back, legs splayed, hair tousled, with a contented look on your face.

I love mornings like this when I can watch you sleep. When the worry lines from your everyday work routine have dissolved and your brow is relaxed. On days like this I want to gently kiss you from the tip of your toes to the top of that often furrowed brow and let you know how much I care. I could count the amount in kisses.

I continue to squeeze the moisture out of my hair with a hand towel, as I study your pose and let my eyes move down over your half covered chest. They drift still further down as I brush the few tangles from my auburn hair and linger at your long legs. I love your legs. I love laying my body along them on a cold winter's night, feeling your heat, as you feel my mouth caressing your most tender parts.

I love running my red painted nails up and down them, lightly scratching the surface of your skin until goose-bumps appear and I hear you moan with pleasure. I love massaging your inner thighs, making you anticipate what my next move might be. I love the feel and scent of you, the texture of your skin. I crave your closeness. Just thinking about touching you makes my body tingle and as I stand there I hear a very soft moan. I realize it came from me and smile as I lay the brush on the dresser. My blue silk robe has managed to slide open and I stand there naked underneath, except for a pair of high-cut black cotton panties, trying to decide what to do.

It's becoming late in the day and I know you'll be rising soon, so why not wake you in a sensual fashion? Your toe peeks invitingly out of the sheets and I bend to kiss it lightly. You stir a little in your sleep again and a little smile tugs at the corners of your mouth, so I decide the time is right.

I raise the corner of the sheet and begin placing soft sensuous kisses along your toes and onto the top of your foot. My hands massage your arches as I move upward, keeping count of the kisses I bestow to every inch of your warm flesh ... 10 ... 11 ... 12 ...

You begin to stretch and groan a little, slowly becoming aware of my attentions, and a smile lights up your face as you open your eyes to see me disappearing under the end of the comforter. 'Mmmm, what's this, breakfast in bed?' I hear you murmur. I stop to chuckle, then continue kissing and counting ... 19 ... 20 ... 21 ... 'Why are you counting?' you say in a sleepy voice as you stretch a little more. 'I want to see how many kisses it takes to get to your mouth', I say with a smile you can't see.

I begin to vary the touch of my lips on your skin, sometimes brushing lightly across your skin, sometimes sucking your flesh into my mouth or nibbling gently. Your body jumps slightly with the aggressive touches and relaxes with the gentle ones. You never know what to expect as I creep closer to the place where your legs meet your torso. The journey so far has yielded 34 kisses and I have a long way to go before my lips meet yours.

You reach over to the night table and grab a stick of gum, crumpling the paper and tossing it towards the waste paper basket. You miss your mark by mere inches because I picked the very moment that you tossed it, to kiss you on the most tender spot on your body. You lift the covers to allow me a little air and comment that I seem to have gotten off track. My kissing line has stopped momentarily while I explore the regional terrain.

I smile, an evil little grin. 'I couldn't resist', I pant as my mouth eagerly takes you in. 'I love a girl with a weak will,' you chuckle between moans. Your body undulates beneath me, slipping your hard member deep into my mouth, across my hungry tongue. You throw the comforter back, leaving only the light sheet covering me.

My robe has long since slipped off, exposing my bare shoulders and ample breasts. You keep the sheet over me delighting in the feel of the actions within. My breasts rub lightly against your warm inner thighs, just above your knees and you feel my firm shoulders against the palms of your hands.

You raise one foot and rub against my bended legs, moving up and down my outer thigh. My body is so aroused by your touch I begin to moan softly, creating a vibration that moves up your shaft and deep into your groin. You move your foot to the warm place between my legs and begin to gently brush against my panties. It creates a tickling sensation and raises me to yet another erotic plateau.

I hear you softly mumble something, but it's lost among the sheets. Words aren't important. We communicate now by touch. I only want to know that I'm pleasing you and that becomes clear in the chorus of moans we create together. You're obviously pleasing me too.

My hips begin to pulse against your foot and you push your toes against the fabric, running them under the side from time to time, exciting me more and more, teasing me. I want your hands and your mouth on me but your needs come first. I feel your urgency growing with each stroke of my tongue and feel your body tensing under me.

My hands work your flesh expertly, and you lift yourself to me, driving deeper with each upward thrust until you explode against the back of my throat. Your body quivers in my hands until you finally rest your derrière back on the mattress.

I continue my kissing and counting beginning at the top of

your thigh with number 35 ... 36 ... 37 ... Upwards my mouth roams, biting, sucking, my tongue taking tiny licks of your warm skin, damp with the efforts of our lovemaking. I love the musky, masculine smell of you, love to feel the contours of your muscle fibres running under the surface of your skin, love the salty taste of you ... 40 ... 41 ... 42 ...

'Mmmm, what a wonderful way to wake up,' you say, smiling gently as you search my eyes. 'What's the occasion?'

'You just looked too delicious to pass up,' I say teasingly, throwing in a wink for good measure. You chuckle softly and your hands run slowly up my back and into my hair ... 44 ... 45 ... Your hands press my mouth against your nipple and I linger there for a few moments, circling it with my tongue and flicking lightly. My mouth surrounds it, tugging gently, sucking and nibbling until you begin to moan again.

My hands roam freely about your torso following the muscles from point to point. Massaging firmly, then tickling softly, wooing the nerve endings into a response. Your body seems alive with sensation and I begin to feel another erection against my inner thigh.

I look up into your eyes and raising one eyebrow say, 'Mmmm, feels like Wee Willie Winkie wants to play again.' You throw your head back into the pillows and let out a loud, body-shaking laugh. I begin to giggle with you and lay my body on top of yours. I love to feel the vibrations move up from your body through mine as you laugh. It's the thing I love most about you. Your sense of fun, your laughter and the way you let out a little gasp when caught off guard.

When the laughter subsides I begin to count again ... 46 ... 47 ... 48 ... I move up your chest towards your neck. I love to kiss your neck and breathe against it until it tickles you and sends shivers up your spine. My tongue reaches out to draw your earlobe into my mouth just as I count ... 55 ... 56 ... and I suck the velvety soft flesh there. You love the tingles it gives you and moan in reply to my whispered plea to feel you inside me.

Suddenly, you roll me over onto my back and your large smooth chest is over me. You reach down and cup my warm mound in your large hand, massaging in a sensual motion. Electrical currents shoot up my spine and my body arches up under you in response. Your fingers slide under the edge of my panties and you feel the soft smooth skin, laid bare by my razor.

You feel the tingles inside your chest and groin area as your fingers become moist, slipping deeper and deeper inside. My breath catches in my throat and I gasp with uncontrolled ecstasy. My hands push down on the waistband of my panties, begging you to remove them. You oblige with one quick stroke of your strong hands and I hear the fabric strain as if it will tear.

My excitement builds higher as you become more and more aggressive and your hands spread my legs to allow you access between them. You stop momentarily, looking deep into my blue eyes and begin to kiss a similar spot on my neck, where I left off on yours.

You count as you kiss across my cheek and position your body between my legs ... 57 ... 58 ... 59 ... The last number is muffled as our lips meet and your long hard shaft slowly slides upward into me, causing a long deep moan from us both. The counting is complete.

Dorothy, 28, computer technician

There is silence in the still of the night. I am anxious, excited and nervous all at the same time. His letter said he would be arriving a little before dawn. It has been so long since I had held him, felt him, kissed him. I have been waiting for this moment for a long time.

We have written to each other every day, saying how much we miss each other and long for each other's touch.

I am daydreaming of how good it will feel to have him home again. I long to make passionate love to him. We always have great sex but I know it will be even better this time.

I run a warm bath and slip out of my robe. I can't resist the urge to touch myself, dreaming it is him touching me. As I am about to climax, the bathroom door opens. There he is, looking better than I had dreamed. He walks over and kisses me gently on the lips. He begins to undress slowly and climbs into the bath with me. He grabs my head and begins kissing me profusely all over my face and neck. He then moves to my nipples taking one in his mouth and rubbing the other with his hand.

I am moaning in pleasure, professing my love for him and begging him to make love to me. I move into his lap and begin riding him. First starting out slowly until I can't stand it anymore and then begin riding with all my might, pushing my pelvis onto his hard cock. He knows I am about to climax and takes me off him and carries me into our bedroom. He has missed everything about me and wants to make this night never end. He lays me on the bed and begins kissing me everywhere. When he gets to my hot spot, I am soaking wet and he begins slowly licking it from top to bottom. I am beginning to feel light-headed. He licks slowly and sticks his finger into my vagina.

After I start moving my pelvis he begins licking harder with two fingers inside me. He knows I am about to burst so he lets me come, burying his face in it and tasting my juices. I scream and my body begins to spasm with pleasure. He lays back on the bed and tells me how much he loves me and has missed me and that he thinks about me non-stop and never wants to leave me again.

I move on top of him and start kissing his neck and mouth. I lick my way down to his nipples and then down to his bulging hardness. I lick his cock from top to bottom, making him beg me to put it in my mouth. My mouth moves over the top of it and I let him feel my breath and the warmth of my mouth as I consume him. I suck with all my might, making him come all inside me. I feel his warm juice slide down my throat.

I wake up alone.

Michelle, 25, nurse

Since I am between lovers and celibate at the moment, my fantasies consist mainly of things I miss about my exes and having sex with them. I love having my breasts licked and sucked, also having someone go down on me.

There's a doctor I fantasize about a lot, a guy I had a relationship with. The ultimate scene is him saying: 'Take off your clothes.'

He was incredibly sexy and we had great sex, and when it was over he got up and left. I was semi-devastated but semi-happy to be alone reliving it. The only difference is in my fantasy, I am the one leaving and he is begging me to stay.

Helena, 29, personnel manager

I was involved with a man for five years before we broke up last year. While together, we wrote love and sex letters to each other. After we broke up, he sent me this letter. I often take it out and masturbate to it, pretending that what he has written is really happening:

'Just thought I would get right into it ... I would love to nibble stiffening nipples feeling them grow within my mouth soft and gentle at first, then rougher, the wetter you get. I would love to have you straddle my wet hot tongue ... pulling those panties to the side and sinking down the length of my delicious tongue meeting you, lip to lip. I would then run the underside of my tongue along your entity, again gently first till your pussy was scorching hot and your lips swollen with nectar ... I would milk that hot clit bobbing up and down your stiff hot clit letting my teeth run down the sides and back to the very tip, giving it a hot nibbling while wrapping my entire mouth around your pussy, flickering my tongue deep inside you. I would savour your clitoral hood until you closed your eyes and began to fuck this wild hot tongue until you could not stand it. Yeah, I have been thinking of you.'

Emma, 27, postgraduate student

I am alone masturbating when I think I hear the front door open. I am feeling so good that I ignore it. Enjoying the sensations my fingers are giving me, I keep my eyes closed as I hear someone enter the room.

'Emma, are you awake?'

It's my ex-boyfriend. We'd broken up the week before and I remember that I had agreed to give him the things he'd left at my flat back this morning. Somewhere in the back of my head floats up the thought, 'He must still have the key to get in.'

In reality, I leapt up, threw on a dressing down and pretended I had slept late. But when I think about the moment now, I dream that I moan softly, my fingers bringing my orgasm closer. He approaches the bed, pulling the covers off. His hands slides down to between my legs, feeling my clitoris pulsating away. He leans down and sucks my clitoris. The orgasm comes racing over me, my clitoris driving against his mouth. We spend the rest of the day making love.

Felicia, 33, mother

My main thing is based on something that actually happened with an old boyfriend. Only now I imagine it is my husband who I did these things with. We are out at dinner and acting really sexy, blowing each other kisses. Later, at a dance club, we can't keep our hands off each other. On the way home, we stop twice for a couple of back seat quickies. When we finally get home, we make love on the balcony, under the stars, for hours, even though it's raining. We still go to the dance club, but we never make it past 10 o'clock before we are forced – by lust – to leave.

Andrea, 30, waitress

My last boyfriend – whom I'll call Henry – was an incredible lover, much better than my current boyfriend. This is the fantasy I sometimes slip into when we are making love.

I imagine Henry and I meet up in a restaurant after we've broken up. The force of his kiss takes me by surprise since he was the one to end it with me. We are both overcome by passion and decide to skip dinner. He leads me to his car and we sink into the soft seats. My heart races as we head towards his flat. I know this is wrong for me, but I can't help myself. We're kissing against his front door as he fumbles with the lock. Our tongues explore, pressing into each other's mouths.

As we head to the bedroom, I notice pictures of a woman. 'My new girlfriend,' says Henry, smiling challengingly, expecting me to react with tears. But knowing that it's me, my body, that Henry wants, I simply shrug and drag him into the bedroom.

He pushes me gently down on to the bed, turning me over ... his hand reaches for the zipper on my dress. I can feel it slowly sliding down my back, his warm hands sliding between the sides of the open dress, caressing my skin. His hot breath caresses me as he kisses a trail down my back. He undoes my bra and slips his hands underneath me, massaging my breasts. His hands pull gently at the dress, sliding it down my body. His mouth comes down in the small of my back, tongue tasting my sweat. He goes lower, pulling off my panties, tongue licking between my cheeks, reaching between my legs. As the dress slides to the floor, he rolls me over slowly, exposing my body. His mouth comes down hard on my mouth for a moment, then slides slowly over me. His tongue flicks softly into my belly button as he moves slowly down. His hands spread me wide, mouth covering me.

I feel exquisite pleasure as he sucks me deep into his mouth. My orgasm takes swiftly, flooding him with my juice. He holds me fast, savouring my taste. I hear him unzip his trousers and feel myself wanting him inside of me. His erection is massive. He spreads my legs wide and gently presses forward, filling me slowly. I gasp as he pushes hard into me. He pulls slowly out, rubbing the head all around my lips before driving back in. My nipples rub against his chest as he moves in and out and I hear myself moaning louder and louder as he moves faster, pushing me hard against the bed. I feel his pace increase and him growing inside of me. His breath comes fast as his climax takes him. I follow seconds later. As he recovers, I slip him out of me and begin getting dressed, knowing I must go before his girlfriend returns.

Melissa, 25, PA

I'm down at the gym and this really muscley bloke wants to have sex with me. We're both hot and sweaty because he's been lifting weights and I've just done a step class. He peels off my leotard and our sticky bodies touch. I love the hardness of his body. He's really strong, his lovemaking is gentle but very firm. And he's got a lot of stamina. I imagine running my fingers over his rippling muscles and the sight of his arms as they hold him up when he's thrusting on top of me. He's telling me what a wonderful body I have, which isn't true in reality but is in my fantasy.

I've never been with someone who is really muscley. I kind of admire those bodies from a distance but think they're a bit over-the-top.

Lucy, 28, nursery teacher

When Dave and his wife Caroline (my best friend) come to visit, I often think about seducing Dave (I never would). I imagine I am making dinner and Caroline goes to the store to pick up some wine. Dave comes into the kitchen to talk with me and I gently back up against him and rub him as we talk. He gets hard and big. I continue to rub and soon he takes out his penis – it's enormous (Caroline has always said it was but I hadn't realized HOW big) – and starts to work it into me. I lie on my stomach on the kitchen floor and he caresses me and fucks me like a dog. There's not much time, so we both come fast. Caroline returns just as we are straightening our clothes. I hope she doesn't notice our flushed faces.

Anne-Marie, 26, occupational therapist

Being in the presence of a man I find sexually attractive and thinking of him when not in his presence gets me off in a big way. I find myself actually picturing his nude body. Especially his penis and the hair on his chest. I long to feel him with my hands and make love to him, to surprise him with the best blow job he's ever had (giving great oral sex is another fantasy of mine as I always worry about my skill in this).

I have these fantasies daily. Sometimes I include replays of past sexual experiences.

Kathy, 20, student

My fantasy is getting it off with a famous person. Usually it's whomever I have just seen in a movie or a concert. But they have to be a bit wild and dirty. Right now, I'm into Liam Gallagher. I go to a gig and have a ticket to a party backstage. During the course of the evening, I notice him looking at me and finally he comes over and chats me up, he tells me I'm the most beautiful woman he's ever seen and he has to have me. The thrill for me is that he's famous and could have anyone he wants, but he chooses me. He's besotted with me and wants to spend the rest of his life loving me. It's like he's been given a love drug and can't leave me alone. He takes me off to a private room and we have mind-blowing sex.

I also masturbate thinking about being fucked by Green Day, Kurt Cobain and other rock stars.

I'm getting bored with my fantasies and wish I had some new material! Maybe I'll explore pornography – although what I've seen of that isn't exactly a turn-on.

Anonymous

It had been at least five months since I'd engaged in any sort of sexual activity with a man. My friends and I were fantasizing about which celebrity we'd sleep with in a heartbeat. My choice was Russell Crowe.

In my fantasy, I go to a virtual sex store, which is a place where you can have sex with whoever you want. I walk in to a dimly lit room with a counter, a young man working the register, and a sign indicating the cost – $25 an hour. 'Who would you like to have virtual sex with?' he asks. I don't have to think about it. 'Russell Crowe.'

'Oh, he's one of our hottest sellers. Good choice.'

He leads me to a small private room containing nothing but a chair. 'You need to sit down here, and place your arms and hands on the arm rests. I'll set you all up, and when you're done, you can just take off the helmet and leave everything the way it is.'

I sit down in the chair. He pulls the black helmet which was attached to the chair around to the front and puts it over my eyes. I place my arm on the rests, and he moves my hands so they touch the pads on the ends.

'Comfortable?' he asks.

'Yes.' I am breathing hard and my heart is beating very fast.

'Okay, here you go.' I hear him pull some kind of switch, and then the door closes as he leaves the room.

The first thing I am aware of is that I am sitting outside a cafe, with a coffee drink sitting in front of me. It's incredible. Everything I see, hear, and smell is absolutely real. As I sit there looking around, Russell Crowe approaches my table and bends slightly to speak to me. 'Uh, hi,' he says, flashing his trademark smile. 'Do you mind if I sit here?'

'No, not at all,' I tell him. He sits down next to me. The table is so small that our thighs press up against each other. 'I don't normally ask strange women if I can sit with them, but you are so beautiful and sexy that I just had to talk to you for a while. What's your name?'

'Margaret,' I say, breathlessly. He is simply gorgeous.

'Hi, Maggie, I'm Russ. I hope you don't mind me saying this, but I want to fuck you so bad my dick is hard just looking at you ...'

I almost gasp out loud when he says this. I am at a loss for words, but he certainly isn't. He leans close to my ear and whispers, 'Let's get out of here.' I feel his warm breath on my ear. It makes me tingle. We end up on the third floor of a building. On the escalator up, he stands behind me, pressing his pelvis against my ass. I can feel his hard cock through his jeans, so I reach around back of me and began to rub his crotch. He groans and I feel his bulge move. As I apply a bit more pressure, he leans in closer to me and begins to kiss the back of my neck. I melt. By the time we get off the escalator, I am dripping wet.

Immediately, he pushes me up against the wall and kisses me ravenously, his hands exploring my body voraciously. I kiss him back with a passion I haven't felt in what seemed like years.

'Oh God,' I gasp as his hands find my breasts. For a moment, he caresses them both gently, while our kisses become less hurried and more tender. Then, in one swift movement, he grabs the front of my blouse, rips it open and sends buttons flying. Immediately, he pulls the cups of my bra down, exposing my breasts and rock hard nipples. Cupping both breasts in his hands, he lifts them up to his mouth, and begins to suck the small pert mounds of my nipples, alternating from one to the other, circling each one with his tongue. Shivers go up and down my spine, and I moan. Instinctively, I press my crotch against his, wanting to feel him inside of me. I begin fumbling with his belt.

Russell knows exactly what I want. I unfasten his belt and the button on his jeans, he continues to fondle and suck on my breasts. I unzip his pants and am delighted as his hard cock pops out of his pants to greet me, unfettered by briefs or boxers. I grab onto it firmly, stroking up and down. Now it is his turn to moan. When I see that he can't stand it a moment longer, I unfasten my own jeans, and he furiously pulls them down. His fingers go directly to my wet pussy, and feeling my wetness, he brings his hand back up to his mouth, licking off my moisture. He kisses me passionately, and I taste my juices on his tongue. My only mission in life at that moment is to have Russell's cock deep inside of me. I slide to the floor and beckon for him to join me.

As he slips inside of me, I feel like I will climax right away. It's been so long since I've felt like that, and it's wonderful. He pumps slowly at first, using his fingers to massage my clit as he slides in and out of my dripping hole. 'Oh, fuck me hard,' I whisper, 'fuck me, fuck me, fuck me.'

When he senses I am on the brink, he teases me by withdrawing completely, waits a second, then plunges back inside.

I gasp with the force of his entry, feeling his dick touch my innermost parts. His hand never leaves my clit, and within minutes, I am writhing in ecstasy. I feel my pussy contracting around his cock as his driving thrusts become more intense. He is close to coming too, so I wrap my legs around him, pressing him deeper inside. With one more powerful lunge, he groans and I feel all of his muscles tighten. His face becomes contorted with the intensity of his orgasm and he gasps. All at once, he relaxes, and I can feel his weight press against me.

At that moment, my fantasy ends but I am still tingling from the reality of my orgasm.

Lena, 31, mother

When I get tired of my boyfriend Liam, sometimes I do it with Harrison Ford. Harrison and I have had our heavy periods, around the time *Sabrina* came out, when I bought myself some dark lipstick like Julia Ormond's that worked on me like an aphrodisiac, and again during the re-release of the *Star Wars* trilogy. Oh, Han! Save me!

But when Harrison gets into his military-presidential persona, I'm forced to look elsewhere. Like at the DIY shop. The guy who does it for me every time at the hardware store is the least likely candidate for anybody's sexual fantasy. He's the short guy, with the podgy body and the slightly cute but frankly babyish face. He's younger than me by about, oh, 18 years. But there's something magnetic about him that makes me undress in front of him. Lead him into that dusty back room where they keep the cans of avocado green and Pepto-Bismol pink paint and tug down his zipper. Get down on my knees ...

Barbara, 29, PR

Often I have a fantasy related to a recent past experience. For instance, if I've been talking to a hunky guy in my office, I will fantasize about him. My new assistant is a really cute young guy who looks just like the actor Ed Furlong. I'd never want to jeopardize my position or our working relationship by approaching him sexually, but I have these wild fantasies of him bringing me morning coffee – and more – in bed.

Patricia, 35, cook

Naked, I slip under the covers, my hands lightly stroking my body as I lay there thinking about the movie I saw with Brad Pitt last night. My fingers pinch my nipples lightly, then I run the palms of my hands over the hard buds. I can feel the wetness beginning between my legs. I slide a hand over my mound, feeling the smoothness. I slip one finger into my cunt, then bring it back to my mouth, tasting my juices.

I pull a vibrator from under my pillow and work it slowly into my wet slit, imagining it to be Brad's cock. I flip the switch to low and feel the soft pulses deep within my cunt. I lay there, enjoying the sensations, tightening my vaginal muscles around the vibrator. I close my eyes and just lay there, the vibrator bringing me to orgasm.

Mandi, 26, project manager

In your fantasies you can be whatever you want to be – that's why they're so brilliant. In mine, I'm the most beautiful woman in the world. I'm with a bloke who's a cross between Brad Pitt and Albert Einstein – looks and brains – and he's so in love with me he says he'll never let me go. Although we make love, it's not just about sex. It's love of the highest order and the orgasms are sensuous and never ending. He adores me and is totally committed to me, there's no specific scenario – it's more that the feelings he has for me that is the turn-on. In real relationships, I hate feeling insecure and worrying about whether my boyfriend feels the same way about me as I do about them, so I guess I look for those feelings in my fantasies.

Rory, 31, events manager

I'm at Wembley watching Ricky Martin play. He's sex on legs. Suddenly he looks out over the sea of faces, spots me and invites me on stage. Once the gig is over, he takes me back to his room for a night of passion. After he's had me, he calls in the rest of his band and we start over again.

Carla, 32, advertising executive

I like the whole concert and rave atmosphere. All the sweating bodies and the scent of sex in the air. These things turn me on. Here is my latest favourite fantasy: I am at our local and my favourite singer is performing. As he strums his guitar, I'm rooted in my spot, forgetting what time of day it is, even what day it is. I forget that this man is basically a stranger to me. In this moment, he sincerely shows me his soul; his playing is not so extraordinary, though he is very good. No; it's the sweet tones that his guitar makes. The way it resonates in his hands and sings with the voice that he gives it.

My heart soars with those notes, feeling so free and flying. I'm bathed in his sound, and I experience the almost overwhelming intimacy of it all. In that moment, I want to drink this man in. I want to take him completely into me, feeling his passion, his love, his soul. I want to enfold him in my arms, feel his bare chest against my breasts, feel his crotch bulging against my belly, tasting his skin and lips. I want to swim in his eyes and let him explore my body, leaving no crevice or spot undiscovered.

My head is reeling now, and I feel my legs almost give way. He finishes, and looks up. His face is flushed, his lips are parted. He looks like he just left his lover's embrace, and is still in the throes of passion.

He reaches up with one hand and replaces a wayward strand of hair. I imagine myself leaning towards him to kiss him. My breath catches in my throat as I feel his soft lips slightly part, and his tongue lightly brushes my open lips. I respond by opening my lips a little further, and slipping my tongue out to meet his lips. A hand touches my hip, moving down to cup my cheek, while the other goes behind my neck. I move my hands to his shoulders, feeling those smooth muscles under his shirt.

He pulls me close, and I feel his bulge against my belly, pressing with such urgency. My breasts crush into his chest, and he slips his tongue further into my mouth, sweetly but with total determination. I open up to him, my body going soft and melding into him, his lips and tongue bathing my mouth with his wetness. I let my hand wander down his arm to his ass, and gently press and squeeze his cheek.

I'm once again lost in his sweet music, but now I'm his guitar. He's making me. He's playing me. His fingers are stroking and strumming. And my body responds by resonating to his touch, quivering like the guitar strings when strummed. But all songs have to eventually end, and this one is no different.

We pull back and look at each other, our hands lingering on each other's bodies for just a moment, and then they slip back to our sides and to their proper places. What words do we utter now, after such a passionate, spontaneous kiss!

I decide to quietly acknowledge the situation and leave.

'Thanks again. That was wonderful. You make beautiful music.' I reach up and stroke his cheek as our eyes meld into each other.

Tess, 31, credit controller

I made up this fantasy when this guy who looks like George Clooney moved in next door to me a few years ago. We've since become good friends and I don't really think he looks like George Clooney any more, but I still like to use this fantasy when I'm masturbating.

I run into my new neighbour in the lift. He's very cute and looks familiar but I can't place him. He says he's new to the neighbourhood and do I know a good place to get a drink. When I hear his voice, I realize that it's George Clooney.

Very unlike the usual me, I am forward and say, 'My place?'

He takes me up on my offer and comes back to my flat with me. I disappear into the kitchen to mix us some vodka tonics. We sit together on the couch and talk. I am sitting close enough to him to feel the heat from his body. We chat about a range of topics, and we find that we have a fair amount of things in common, including a love for vodka.

The glasses are refilled a couple of times, and the conversation grows a little bolder, dealing more with our sex lives. I mention that I haven't had a boyfriend for a while. He says he can't believe that when I am so unbelievably sexy.

He takes my hand gently and pulls it toward his mouth, turning the wrist up and kissing it lightly at the pulse point. A shiver runs through me, as it's one of my favourite spots. His tongue flicks out, just licking up my arm lightly. A slight moan escapes my lips, although I try to muffle it. I pull him toward me. My mouth covers his, my tongue pressing insistently into his mouth. His arms go tight around me, holding me close as we sit on the couch kissing. His mouth breaks the kiss and slides down my throat, kissing and nibbling as it goes.

I lift my arms as he pulls my top off, over my head. My bra is the next thing to go. His mouth travels over the path of the bra, licking at the marks it's left. His tongue traces a path over the nipples and pulls one gently into his mouth. One of his hands slides down the waistband of my skirt, searching. I can't wait and pull off the rest of my clothing and lie back. He has also undressed. He lies on the floor and I climb on top of him and we make love for the rest of the night.

Diana, 31, social worker

I'm on vacation in Australia with my boyfriend. Except he isn't my boyfriend. He's Mel Gibson. We are exploring the outback and stop for lunch at a rest stop that looks as though it hasn't been used in a while. We sit on a log, legs touching while we eat, hands just touching now and again, stroking an arm or a leg.

Afterward, we decide to take a walk down the trail, exploring a little. The terrain is rough, but the walk is wonderful. The heat is pretty intense so we're glad to come upon a water hole. Huge trees surround the crystal clear water. We don't have suits, but can't resist the cool-looking water. We strip and race to see who will be first. I beat Mel by a hair, splashing into the cooling water. We swim a little, play a lot. We meet in the water, mouths pressing against one another.

We kiss softly at first, tongues probing, fingers wandering. We climb out onto one of the rocks, the sun beating down on us. As our bodies dry, we continue our exploring, slow and unhurried. Mel's fingers trace the lines of my face and my throat. I feel his mouth press against my neck, trailing up to my ear, nibbling slightly. His fingers stroke my shoulders, slipping down slowly to my breasts. He dips a hand into the water, and let some drip onto my breasts. He dips his hand into the water again, this time leaving a trail of water running down my body, approaching my own wetness. His fingers slowly follow the water, fingers pausing around the entrance to my pussy, teasing me a little. One finger slowly pushes in, causing my body to arch against his hand. Another finger slides in, joining the first. His thumb begins to stroke my clit, bringing my first orgasm.

Mel lies back on the warm stone. I position myself over him, sliding him deep inside me. I push down hard and feel him fill me. I begin to move over him, leaning forward, my hair brushing his chest. His hands lift to my breasts, stroking them as we move in rhythm. The sun beats down on us, warming our already hot bodies. We climax together.

brief encounters

Introduction

You're standing on the bus during rush hour and pressed right against you is a dark haired stunner. You feel your bodies rocking together with the motion of the bus. Then suddenly, the object of your desire starts pushing against you. You respond. You both explode in glorious orgasms and then part, without exchanging a word.

Whatever your favourite fantasy is, practically every woman has at some time or another thought about ravishing a gorgeous stranger. Studies show that the nameless fuck tends to be an especially hot fantasy for women because it lets them overcome the guilt and inhibitions that often block arousal and sexual satisfaction for women. Whether it's the sexy man spotted on the street, the waiter at the restaurant where you're out with your boyfriend, the guy next door, or simply a person you conjure up in your imagination, fantasizing about having wild abandoned sex with a total stranger allows you to have the thrill of anonymously indulging your deepest desires. There's no fear of STDs, pregnancy, being in real physical danger, the emotional responsibility of being in a relationship or, if you're already hooked up, getting caught. You don't even have to deal with the rigmarole of getting acquainted or figuring out if you should stay the night. In its place is a man who is always gorgeous, usually consumed with lust and – best of all – dying to pleasure you from head to toe.

Helen, 29, waitress

This is the fantasy I have after I have had an especially hard day. I prepare when I get home. I undress, step into the bathtub and sink into the steamy water. Leaning back and closing my eyes, I feel my body finally relax for the first time in what feels like a month. I rest that way for a while till the water begins to cool too much to be comfortable.

I towel myself dry and slip between the coolness of the sheets on my bed. My mind drifts in a state of half sleep, half wakefulness.

I feel someone quietly crawl into bed next to me. 'Just relax. I know you had one hell of a day. Close your eyes and let me help you sleep,' a voice whispers.

Hands – male? female? – caress my face as fingers lightly massage my temples. I sigh as I drift further away. Barely touching my body, fingertips travel down my neck, across my breasts to the pinkness of my nipples. The tip of my nipple is touched lightly and it hardens. With barely any pressure, I feel it massaged in a circular motion. A slight moan escapes my lips.

I feel the person move lower on the bed and feel each nipple gently sucked between hungry lips. Hands move to my shoulders and down each arm, kneading my tired muscles. Each of my fingers is massaged in slow motion ... I drift for I don't know how long.

The hands return to my breasts, then lower, massaging my waist and stomach. I feel someone kneel between my legs at the foot of the bed. My feet are massaged, including each toe. Expertly, the hands move up my legs. My muscles melt from the touch. Oil is added. I spread my legs willingly as fingers slide down the length of my smooth, shaven lips. Slowly, each crease and fold of my womanhood is stroked and massaged between a thumb and forefinger. My clitoris starts to grow. My wetness mixes with the oil and my hips begin a slow, almost undetectable rhythm.

An index finger is slid inside me, while a thumb continues to massage me. With the other hand, a steady pressure is applied to the top of my mound. My clitoris is fully extended now and gently, a tongue snakes across it. I feel my muscles tighten on the finger which is inside of me. The tongue continues to circle and stroke me.

My breathing becomes more laboured. I can feel my orgasm building. In my dreamlike state, my arousal grows, taking me to new heights. I drift and flow upward with each new sensation. My hips move more earnestly and stroke myself on the fingers still pressing against me.

I am near the edge now. It seems difficult to breathe. My lungs expand as I draw in more oxygen. My back arches, lifting my hips off the bed. My whole body tenses as the first strong spasms overtake me, then I relax and flow.

The body moves with me. Lips suck in my clitoris while the tongue stimulates me further. I feel the contractions of my orgasm begin. I hear myself groan with the sudden release. I float higher as I go over the edge. My muscles squeeze the fingers inside of me.

Each new wave washes over me, releasing the tension and sapping my energy. The spasms weaken in intensity but continue on. I drift for what seems like forever.

Carla, 25, marketing manager

There's a storm raging outside. I'm watching the rain course down the window. Idly, I run my hand up and down my arm, enjoying the contact. Slowly I start stroking my breasts. My nipples harden and I continue to play with them, enjoying the sensation. I slide my fingers through the lips of my cunt. I'm already a little wet. I start massaging my clit and as I get caught up in an orgasm, the lightning flashes and I see a shadow of someone standing in the room. 'Who the hell is that?' I scream.

It's a man, completely soaked. 'Sorry, my car broke down. I knocked but I guess you didn't hear me,' he says. 'I was looking for somewhere to call the auto club. It's a hell of a night out there.' I wonder how much he saw before I saw him. Then I notice he is exactly my type: dark hair, dark eyes, tall, strong jaw. I grab a blanket from the couch and say, 'You look cold. Why don't you get out of those things and wrap this around yourself.'

I turn my back to let him change, but he doesn't realize I can still see him in the mirror. I watch, transfixed. His body is muscular and tanned. 'Done,' he murmurs. I turn and he is standing so close to me that my breasts brush against his chest. I lean forward and kiss him softly. He pushes closer against me, his tongue pressing into my mouth. We move to the couch. He spreads my legs, pushing my dress up my legs. His head lowers to my cunt, fingers spreading me wide, tongue plunging deeply into me. I gasp with pleasure as he brings me quickly to climax, my juices dripping onto his face. I lie there feeling completely satisfied. He kisses me lightly on the lips and leaves.

Christina, 29, photographer

I am with this wild man. He does everything. He kisses me all over – my feet, my neck, inner thighs. He massages my shoulders and back. When we really get into it, he makes me sweat like a football player. It is dripping down my back and he kisses and licks me up and down. I have orgasm after orgasm – it is as if I get energy from a place in my body I never knew about. I have straight hair, but when it's all over, my hair is actually curly.

Anonymous

I'm on the bus home – and there's only me and a gorgeous stranger left on the top deck. He comes over and ravishes me on my seat before getting off at the next stop. Panting, I realize I don't even know his name.

Annette, 27, lifeguard

I've always had a thing for a sauna. The heat and steam brings out not only sweat, but my most base desires. I imagine that I'm at a hotel and it's just after 9pm. I decide to take a quick trip down to the sauna before it closes. I put my towel on the bench and throw some water on the rocks, allowing the steam to flow over me. I sit down on the bench enjoying the heat.

Just as I slip a hand down between my thighs, the door opens. It's a good-looking man in his early thirties. He sits pretty close to me. He turns towards me and says he likes my swimsuit, and reaches out and touches one of my nipples. I gasp with the contact, and pull back slightly. The heat I feel when he touches me is intense. I lean forward and lightly touch the bulge that is now straining against his trunks.

We kiss deeply. He lifts the straps of my suit off, and peels it down my body. He gets down to the lower bench and parts my legs, running his hands up the inside of my thighs, to my waiting pussy. He spreads the lips with his fingers, leans in and runs his tongue along my clit. I begin to climax almost instantly. He continues to lick furiously, and I feel myself building to another climax. As I come over the top, he lifts his head and smiles.

We trade places, and I lift my hands to his cock. I run my fingers lightly over the tip, down the underside and cup his balls lightly. I open my mouth and engulf the tip with it, running my mouth up and down the shaft. I release his cock for a minute and pull each of his balls into my mouth, one at a time. He's rock hard by now. I tell him to get off the bench. We both stand on the floor. I lean forward, putting my hands on the upper bench, presenting my back to him.

'Fuck me, fuck me!' I groan, turning my head to look at him. He comes up behind me and I can feel his body press against mine, his hard cock pressing against my ass. He lowers his hands and opens me up to him as he slides his cock into my wet pussy. I gasp as it fills me. I start to fall, but his strong hands catch me. I feel his hands slide up my body and under my breasts. His fingers slide round and begin to rub my nipples slowly. Then, he begins to move within me, back and forth with enough force to push me forward with each stroke. I slip one hand between my thighs and begin to stroke my clit.

The heat of the sauna and our bodies is making me swoon. I can feel his pace building, and know that his orgasm is close. I cry, 'Faster, faster.' Suddenly he withdraws and his come begins to pulse over my ass. He turns me towards him and the remainder falls on my stomach. As he leans over and kisses my breast, we hear someone coming. We quickly grab our towels and throw them over our bodies. A man from the hotel staff opens the door and tells us the pool will be closing shortly. We struggle back into our suits, and say goodbye. I realize after I get back to my room that I never even knew his name.

Janet, 28, PR manager

I have never simply screwed someone because I was horny. But in my fantasies, I always do. Usually, the man is a stranger whom I've just met at a party or a club. He is so taken with my beauty that he has to have me there, so we slip away to an empty room or even the bathroom. Often we don't even get undressed. I just pull down my panties and he unzips. The main thing is to do it as soon as possible. When I have this fantasy, I can orgasm very quickly – sometimes within seconds from start to finish. I often use it when I know I am about to make love with my boyfriend to get me revved up and in the mood.

Tina, 31, housewife

I imagine that I am a sales clerk, minding the cash register, while a man I can't see hides underneath the counter and rubs my genitals. I'm not in control of the sex. I just allow my body to be available and enjoy the sensations.

Dorothy

We are sitting in a crowded restaurant. You at your table, I at mine. My eyes wander lazily round the room, taking in the sights, sounds and smells of my surroundings. The aroma of fresh tomato sauce and rich spices fill the air, and I breathe deeply and close my eyes. There is romantic music in the background, and its mellow tones caress my ears. The drumbeat makes my heart beat in rhythm, and I once again open my eyes.

This time I notice you, sitting on the far side of the room. Wine glass in hand, slowly and methodically licking your lips, trying to remove all traces of the hot, spicy sauce from the edges of your moustache. Your eyes are clear, and the light from the overhead chandelier makes them twinkle and shine. I detect a bit of mischief there too, and my lips curve into a small, approving smile. I watch your eyes lower slightly to take in the curve of my breasts and lower still seeking the mystery to what lies behind the tablecloth in front of me.

I shift my position in the chair, and swing my legs to the side, crossing them at the knee and revealing a little of my creamy white thigh. You smile and heave a great sigh that lifts your shoulders slightly. I feel a tingle run through my body and wonder what your next move will be.

I can't believe I am flirting across the room with a total stranger. I take the last sip of my wine and I'm about to get up when a waiter asks if I would care to join the gentleman in a private booth for dessert, your treat. He motions toward you and I see you slowly rise. You are tall and lean and you have the most inviting smile on your face. How could I possibly say no?

My heart pounds as I walk in the direction you are headed, behind the waiter. You disappear behind a glass partition, and just as we round the corner I see you disappear through a double door, ornately carved with intricate patterns of leaves and swirls. As we near the room I smell the scent of cinnamon. You are sitting in a small private room full of scented candles. On the table before you are two glasses of white wine and a plate of chocolate-dipped strawberries and fresh whipped cream. I slide into the seat next to you as the waiter closes the door, instructing us to ring if there's anything we need. He bows slightly as he closes the doors behind him, leaving us in the soft candlelight.

I turn to look at you, and you pick up your glass and raise it slightly in my direction saying, 'Here's to the lovely lady and getting to know her better.' I smile and reach for my glass, taking a long, slow sip. The wine coats my lips and you watch as my tongue circles their soft, pink form, being careful not to miss a drop.

On impulse you bend quickly forward and put your mouth over mine, and we kiss passionately, deeply for the first time. The kiss lasts a long time and we are both surprised at how comfortable it feels, like we've done this before many times – and yet we've only just met.

You set down your glass and then reach for mine, placing it on the table in front of me. You slide your chair back and turn my chair to face you. Your eyes search mine, and you slide your fingers through my silken hair, pulling my mouth to yours. We kiss urgently, and I find myself rising from my seat and sliding into your lap, straddling your legs. Your hand is immediately drawn up my thigh as you pet that warm place between my legs, making me sigh and moan at the touch of your expert fingers. My fingers have found your nipples through your shirt and I rub them gently and roll them between my finger tips. My tongue slips quickly into your mouth and plays around yours.

I sense the hunger in your kiss, and slowly begin to unbutton my blouse, revealing my smooth, firm breasts to your waiting lips. You kiss the curves of my soft tits as your tongue reaches down over the edge of my lacy bra, seeking the tender nipples. You pull the lace back with your fingertips releasing my pink nipple as you suck it deep into your mouth, rolling the tip of your tongue around the erect flesh. I lean my head back and moan softly, afraid someone might hear us. Your fingers trace the edge of my panties as my hands wander down your buttons, and I open your shirt to reveal your strong chest.

My hands continue downward and I slowly lower your zipper releasing the pressure you feel. Your hard member pushes against the material of your shorts, and I slide my fingers in and gently pull it through. My fingers gently trace along it, and I let out a deep moan as I realize its length and feel your firm, juicy tip with my thumb. My tongue probes the end of yours, as my fingertips circle your soft head, pushing deeper and deeper into the juicy flesh. I feel you twitch and throb with each stroke, and I know you're imagining it's my tongue doing the work.

Suddenly and without warning you slide two fingers deep into me. I gasp and then make a deep purring noise like a contented cat having a stretch. Your fingers work in and out rhythmically as your thumb circles and excites my hard, sensitive clit. My fingers are still working on your tip as I firmly grip your shaft with my other hand and begin to stroke up and down slowly.

You look into my eyes and we exchange smiles. Then my eyes lower to your erect shaft and I groan with pleasure at the sight of it in my hand. My tongue reaches out to moisten my eager lips. 'Mmmmm, I want to taste you,' I say in a deep sensual tone, and you groan softly at the thought of it.

I gently remove myself from your manipulations and sink to my knees between your legs, your hard cock still in my hands. I stop my work on you and just hold your shaft loosely in my hand. Then I look up and deep into your eyes, and watch them widen as I reach out to gently suck the dribbling cum from the head. I let it pop back out of my mouth, and tickle you with the tip of my tongue a few times before sucking it in again and letting your tip slide across the roof of my mouth to the back of my throat. You lean back in the chair and a long, deep, moan escapes you.

The waiter knocks quietly on the door and asks if everything is to your satisfaction. You reply with a 'Yes' and ask that we not be disturbed. The waiter complies and you direct your attention back to the rise and fall of my silky auburn hair in your lap. You stroke my head and shoulders and arched back, squirming in your chair. My mouth feels so good on you, and your mind is a million miles away, but I'm with you in a soft romantic place, far from the rest of the world.

You moan gently and sigh deeply as I work on your tender flesh, and soon you feel the pressure build up in your groin and you feel you are about to explode. I take one last deep draw from you and feel your creamy load fill my mouth. 'Mmmmm' ... so smooth and sweet, like a warm milkshake. I wait until every last drop has left you and your once hard shaft becomes soft and limp. I lick you gently and then stand up leaning over you to kiss you tenderly.

You rise to meet my mouth and press my body into you. Your mouth wanders down my neck and across the rise of my breasts and you ease me up onto the strong, solid table. You reach down and slip my panties off and then slide my legs up over your shoulders. My back arches in anticipation, and you pause to reach for one of the strawberries. You hold it to my lips and I take a bite. You dip it into the whipped cream and squeeze the juice from it with your fingertips, letting it drip down the newly shaved lips of my ripe, juicy pussy.

I feel the cool drops as they come in contact with my skin and disappear into my pink folds. You look at me with an evil smirk and say, 'Oh gee, sorry. Let me clean that up for you,' and I watch as you run your tongue up my slit and probe inside for the juices hidden there. You lick and suck my tender skin and make me ache for your tongue to enter me further. My hips begin to gyrate to the sound of the muted music, and I moan softly with each careful stroke.

You slide up the length of my slit to my tender clit, and flick it lightly with each passing, driving me more and more crazy with pleasure. 'Mmmmmmm ... unhhhhhhhhhhh .... ooooooooooooooowwwww! That feels disgustingly good. You've spoiled me for any other man. God you're good.'

You raise your head, smile and go back to searching for all the sensitive spots, and you find them one by one. You bring me to the brink over and over, backing off just before climax and beginning again. You start the long slow climb again and then just before I'm about to peak you slide up and into me with your rock hard shaft. I feel every inch of you as you enter, and my body quivers as I realize you're close to orgasm yourself.

You move quickly at first, and then slow down to feel my muscles pulsating around you. I sit up and grip your hot, fleshy ass with my hands pushing you deep into me and we explode together. Shivering with sheer ecstasy at the sensations that take over our bodies. We hold each other close, and I put my head against your chest as I take in your musky scent. You smell so delicious, I want to devour you all over again.

You finally reach down and cup my breast, returning it to the lacy confines of my bra, and begin to fasten the buttons on my blouse. I look questioningly into your eyes and you say. 'I think we should continue this over coffee, at my place.' I grin widely and you bend to give me a peck on the mouth, then raise one of the strawberries to my lips and rub the juice across it. Your tongue gently licks it from me, and I open my mouth and take a juicy bite.

You watch as I slowly chew the ripe berry, licking my lips now and then. As you fasten the last button of your rumpled shirt, you say, 'Hurry, I want those lips on me again. I'm getting hard just thinking about it.' I reach down and stroke your hard member through your pants and whisper in a very sexy voice, 'Patience, darling, I plan to make all your dreams come true, tonight.'

You take my hand and we leave what I have now dubbed my favourite restaurant.

Margaret, 28, teacher

I had a very conservative childhood. My parents thought I should be a virgin until I got married (hah!). Their attitude made me feel guilty about masturbating and even having sexual fantasies. I only recently admitted to my lover that I ever masturbated (he doesn't know that I still sometimes do it). I usually think about the same thing while masturbating:

I am alone in a room. Then arms engulf me. His smell invades my being. His warmth touches me in a way I hadn't felt in a very long time. My heart beat wildly in my chest. My breath is coming in almost ragged spurts. He grabs my shoulders and turns me around, pulling me into his body. My breath catches in my throat as his mouth and tongue finds mine, searching and probing. His hands slide down my back slowly to my ass, and he parts my cheeks and slides his hand in between, against the wet material. His erection is pressing into my belly with considerable force, and he is obviously as aroused as I am.

He slides his hands around to my belly and leans his chin on my shoulder. I let my hands meet his, and our fingers interlace. I like the way he feels, pressed up against me like that. It is warm and comforting and sweet and sexy and ... and everything. More than anything, it is wonderful. Just plain wonderful. I draw in a breath and close my eyes, trying to download the experience into my senses for all time.

His hands slide around my hips and rests on the cheeks, and I let my hands slip to his chest, feeling his hair and muscles beneath my gently teasing fingertips. For blissful minutes, I just explore his chest and stomach and nipples, tracing sometimes, entwining at other times, kneading some other times.

He is beginning to move his hips against me in an almost imperceptible motion. I kiss his sternum, then turn my attention to his hard right nipple, licking and sucking gently. His cock stiffens even more against me, and my body responds to this with harder tits and a wetter pussy. I move my mouth over to his left nipple, and a long, soft moan escapes his throat, almost bypassing his mouth. The only sound is our heavy breathing and occasional moans.

I continue touching and kissing his chest and nipples, then move upward to his neck. I lick his Adam's apple with a broad flat tongue, eliciting more soft, bestial sounds from him. I nibble and suck, and his hips suddenly buck under me. He shoves deep within me and uses his hand to touch my clitoris. His strokes are maddeningly soft and slow, while his thrusts are deep and fast. The combination brings me to orgasm, and as my clitoris spasms against him, he comes too. I feel his warm spunk flow into me and down my legs as he withdraws, both of us breathless and speechless.

Lucy, 28, physiotherapist

I sometimes go through the whole process – from helping a man undress to the final orgasm – all in my mind. My imagination is pretty good and I can 'feel' hands caressing me – a tongue on my clitoris, etc.

In one of my favourite fantasies, I am trapped in a burning house when a hunky fireman shows up. He is calm, controlled and completely gorgeous. He sweeps me off my feet and carries me out of the house. When we are safe, I give him oral sex out of gratitude for saving me. Then we have passionate sex.

Natalie, 29, public relations executive

This is based on a flirtation I actually had. I am flying home from Miami, Florida, to London and standing in the aisle talking to a few fellow passengers when I feel this hand on my back and heard this amazing voice say, 'Sweetheart, don't move.' I look around to see this incredibly handsome flight attendant pushing a cart. We spend the entire flight talking to each other, and he invites me to his layover hotel for lunch. I run home after my nine-hour flight, dress in my most appealing clothes, and go to his room. Lunch waits while I experience the sweetest, most mind-blowing sex of my life.

Jenny, 30, graphic artist

Stuck in traffic while driving home in the car the other night, I slid my hand under my skirt, allowing my thoughts to drift ... I look around at my fellow drivers and wonder what is flashing through their minds ... are they thinking of boring things like what to have for dinner, work tomorrow, bills unpaid? Or is there someone else out there, sliding his hand over the erection pressing against his trousers? I see a rather handsome man in the car next to me and I draw him into my fantasy. Using my cell phone, I call him, somehow knowing the number to dial. When he answers, I whisper, 'You're so sexy. I want to see you pleasuring yourself.' He looks startled for a moment and then he smiles, his arm moving slowly over his hard erection, fingers stroking himself lightly. His eyes close slightly and his lips part as he breathes in and out. His hand runs up under his shirt, fingers stroking his stomach, and his chest, touching a nipple lightly. His hands pull at his belt, needing to release his erection. I can see the red-violet head of his cock, pushing upwards.

He brings his fingers to his mouth, wetting them, then grips his erection. As his hands slide slowly over the shaft, my fingers press under my panties, sliding into my wetness. The traffic is starting to move, so I finish quickly. As the car with the handsome man pulls forward, he smiles at me. Perhaps we did enjoy a fantasy together ...

Anonymous

I am a female executive in an import/export firm. Previously the only females in this business were secretaries. But I came in with a business school education and due to that (and the fact that I am very aggressive and competitive) I am now almost at the top of the organization. In fact (and this has a lot to do with this story) I have a private office and a secretary, Julie. Julie keeps things in order and handles administrative chores for me.

I often read a local newspaper that has, among many other features, a rather amazing set of classified personal ads. Some categories are for the usual service you find in almost any paper – educational, typing, almost anything. But this paper has sexually explicit ads in categories like Men Seeking Women, Men Seeking Men, Women Seeking Men, and Women Seeking Women. There are categories which tend to be a bit wilder like Couples, Transgender, and Anything Goes. I read these personals frequently and get turned on by many of them since they can be very erotic and focus on 'kinky' behaviour. I had never acted on any of them until I read the following ad in *Anything Goes*:

'You're a woman with a sense of adventure, daring, and a private office. This cute White Male will give oral pleasure while you take calls.'

That really turned me on. The thought of a guy going down on me while I took phone calls stirred me up, and that became my favourite masturbation fantasy. I read the well-worn page whenever I wanted a sexual charge.

In my fantasy, I have contacted the box number and the writer of the ad has called me. He sounds like a nice guy and very matter-of-factly tells me that he really likes to perform oral sex on women, that he is very good at it, and that the office setting turns him on. He says it would be fun and exciting for both of us. He will come as 'Mr. Brown' on some pretext at 2pm on the following Wednesday. I feel that I might be doing something stupid and risky, but I am so turned on that I feel compelled to make the appointment.

When getting dressed Wednesday morning I wonder what to wear to get my pussy licked and sucked. I put on a black lace garter belt, and very nice long black stockings – very sexy. Then I put on my best black panties, which could be slipped off while leaving the garter belt and stockings in place.

It seemed crazy to be dressing for this sort of thing, but I am in a state of sexual arousal higher than anything I have felt before. As the clock approaches 2pm, I am nervous, but the usual phone calls and paperwork thankfully take my mind off the coming adventure. 'Mr. Brown' arrives five minutes before the appointed time. My secretary announces his arrival and I say to let him in. He is in his mid-thirties, dressed in a business suit, very handsome. We spend a few minutes in small talk, and then he says he is here to eat my pussy and that we ought to get to it. I nod weakly. He reminds me that it turns him on for me to continue to take business calls while he is giving me pleasure. He tells me to sit sideways in my chair and then he gets on his knees in front of me. He tells me to just lean back and enjoy, while he would take care of giving me what I craved. He has me pull my skirt up and then both of us get my panties down below my knees. Then I just lean back and enjoy an expert giving me the best sexual experience I have ever had.

Some men perform oral sex on a woman reluctantly, only to please their partner – not him! He clearly enjoys the smell and taste of cunt. My pussy is already wet. He uses his tongue on my pussy lips, licking softly and going all the way to the clit. I have a large clit that protrudes when I am aroused. He brings me the edge of an orgasm by using his talented tongue on my bud. Then he brings me over the edge by sucking on it, softly at first and progressively harder and faster. I come with an explosion that rocks my entire body. Just then the phone rings!

It's an indescribable feeling – breathing hard and wanting to moan, and having to talk to a customer on the phone at the same time. But it's also very exciting, getting my pussy serviced while the customer has no idea of what was going on. And, of course, there is the thrill of doing something so 'forbidden' and escaping detection. I'm sure the caller thinks I am very distracted for some sort of mundane reason but has no idea of what is really happening.

I have two more orgasms during the remainder of our time together. 'Mr Brown' just keeps sucking up my juices. There is one more call during this session, from the company president. I manage to handle that call but he must also notice what seems like distraction on my part.

Thirty minutes after my guest's arrival, I have been licked and sucked like never before in my life, and my pussy is soaking wet. I wipe my pussy off with some Kleenex and pull the panties up. Then the skirt comes down, and I am the corporate executive again. 'Mr. Brown' says that he has satisfied his urges and asks how I feel. I respond truly, that it has been great for me. We agree to have him visit me the following week, and I call Julie to schedule 'Mr. Brown' again for a $^1/_2$ hour appointment the following week.

Paula, 31, broker

My fantasies lately tend to be about this guy I know through work. He's in his late forties, very tall, and I find him extremely sexy. So the fantasy is that we're finally alone together and our eyes meet and we kiss passionately and he tells me that he's crazy about me and thinks I'm beautiful and we have this fantastic sex – like premarital sex – long and incredibly exciting and endless and orgasmic.

Wendy, 35, dentist

My friend Jane has asked me to house-sit and watch her cat while she and her family are away. I am in the living room reading when there is a knock on the door. The man at the door is glistening with sweat and panting slightly – he has obviously been running. My heart skips a beat, because he is so incredibly sexy in his little running shorts and sweat-soaked T-shirt. His legs are muscular, but fleshy.

I notice the bulge in his shorts, and he notices me noticing. As I look up into his eyes, he asks, 'Is Janey home?'

When I tell him the whole family is away, he asks, 'Can I come in for a quick drink of water?' I move aside and he walks in and heads straight for the kitchen. He obviously knows his way around. I suddenly realize that Janey is having an affair and this is her lover.

I follow him. He turns and before I can say a word, his mouth is on mine, his arms are around my body, and my breasts are being crushed into him.

I gasp with pleasure. His tongue slides in and around my mouth. His hands caress first my sides, then my ass, then move up to find my ready breasts. They knead and flick while his tongue moves down to my neck, where he starts lightly biting me. I let my head fall backwards and moan, my hand caressing his ass and slipping under the hem of his shorts to find his sweet, bare skin. My fingers probe into his ass and caress him deeply. He groans in response.

He pulls my T-shirt up just enough to get his mouth on my boobs, and he begins a very loud and passionate sucking. I actually climax, it's all so intense. 'Your breasts are bigger than Janey's,' he whispers.

I feel a heat in the pit of my belly and sex whose equal I had never felt before. I am already panting and sweating when he takes my hand and leads me upstairs. Again, he seems to know the way.

When we enter the room our clothes are off in seconds flat. He caresses me all over and then inserts a finger up me. 'Mmmm, juicier than Janey too,' he says. 'Now let's see if you're tighter.' He climbs on top of me and we both explode.

Anonymous

This is a fantasy about a missed opportunity on my recent holiday to Crete. The hotel I stayed in was away from almost everywhere. So most nights, my girlfriends and I hung around the hotel's club. They had a nightly show. One of the dancers caught my eye immediately.

He wasn't very tall, but he had a beautiful body. When the show ended, the music kept playing for anyone who wanted to dance. I headed towards 'my dancer' and asked him to dance. He had dark eyes and a sexy accent and smiled as he took me in his arms.

The song being played had a slow beat, and he pulled me close to him. I could feel the heat of his body as we moved together. The song ended, and I made a move to return to my seat.

'Stay,' he whispered.

I didn't, but now I wish I had.

I imagine that we spend the rest of the night dancing. When the music stops for the night, we keep on dancing to our own inner beat. Spiros – that was his name – takes me in his arms, kissing me softly at first, then just a little harder. Our bodies press against one another. His mouth trails over my face and my neck, the heat bringing moans from my mouth. He pulls my dress over my head, leaving me standing in my panties.

His mouth lowers to my breasts, licking them. His hands caress my breasts, cupping them as his tongue flicks against my nipples. My knees feel weak as his tongue caresses lower on my body. He lowers me to the ground, sitting me on a chair, kneeling between my legs, pulling my panties from me easily.

His fingers stroke my body, slowly dipping into my pussy. He pushes them in and out of me, driving me wild. His tongue joins in giving me pleasure as it circles my clit, then moves to my clit, bringing cries of pleasure from me as my orgasm takes me.

I start clawing at his clothes, tearing them from his muscular body. When I get to his hard penis, I lean forward and draw him into my mouth, feeling his pulsing shaft. My hands slide around his hard body, pulling him closer to me, feeling his hardness fill my mouth.

He cries out in his language. We slide to the floor and I feel him push deep within me. My legs and arms grip him as we grind in passion. We come together in a screaming climax.

We spend the next two weeks of my holiday dancing and fucking every night. When I fly home, I know I'll never see him again, but he's given me with the most satisfying holiday I've ever had.

Mary, 35, personnel officer

I am happily married. But sex has become boring after 10 years. Recently, I've been visiting sex chat lines. Sometimes I am a 15-year-old girl, sometimes I pretend to be a young man. Entering a zone where I can flirt with someone unknown and never meet them allows a sexual freedom that makes all parts of me tingle with desire. The Internet has opened new doors.

In this fantasy, I am logging on, already hot and sticky from anticipation when the sound 'You've Got Mail' clicks on my computer. I click on the mailbox and a picture starts to form on the page. First, I see feet, then legs, then, oh my, I think' and my heart starts to race. This one is handsome. At the same time, I start getting a barrage of questions on line: 'Well? What do you think? Am I OK? Want to play? If you think that bulge in my pants is fake, it is not. I'm 7 inches of pure cock. Wanna fuck?'

If he were here, I'd probably fuck him right on the spot, but this seems too weird. Then he types some more: 'What are you wearing? Touch yourself.'

I do not even know this person. He doesn't even know my name. Names seem to not be important. I sit there for a second debating whether I want to continue. 'How would he know if I were touching myself?' I muse.

'I'm wearing a light blue Victoria's Secret teddy,' I type in, squeezing my thighs because I am definitely feeling a rush to my pussy. I know if I touched myself, I would be very, very, wet.

'Oh yeah. I'm very hard baby. I'm all hard cock right now, sitting in my boxers jumping out to meet you. If I were with you, my tongue would be licking your swollen pussy lips.'

'Mmmmm,' I type. 'I can feel you touching me.'

'Look at my eyes. Look at the picture and focus on my green eyes. I'm moving down your chest now, kissing your neck, your breasts, don't type, just listen, circling each nipple with my tongue, you taste so good. I'm making my way down to your belly, to your pubic bone, nuzzling my nose in your fuzz, smelling you, tasting you, do you like that? Do you like when a man goes down on you?'

I can barely breathe. I read the words and my breath quickens. How it would feel in his arms, the warmth, the strength.

He continues: 'My tongue is on your thighs, I'm outlining your pussy lips and licking the inside of your crack. Tasting your nub, nibbling on it lightly, as you start to quiver and spurt. I love tasting the clear liquid coming out of you as you squirt, ohmigod, you taste so good!'

There is nothing for a minute and my hands are paralysed. I know I should type something back but I can't. All I can feel his tongue on my clit. I feel my orgasm start to build.

'Take two fingers and put them inside you. Push them deep inside you,' he types. Feel your wetness. Feel the dripping onto your palm. Rub yourself until you're hard.'

I start reaching inside my jeans and with two fingers, I follow his command. I am so wet. I haven't been that wet in so long with my husband that it scares me. My body relaxes as I slump down into the chair lost in the ecstasy of sex, of masturbation, enjoying each touch and each feel; I read the words on my screen: 'Yeah baby, I know you're touching yourself. You're silent. I'm going to make you come. You're going to come for me, baby, I want you to take your fingers and squeeze your clit. Squeeze it tight while your rub your juices on it, back and forth until you feel you're going to explode. Think of my head down between your legs with my chin rubbing your clit. Think of me lapping your sweet pussy juices and feeling the quivering of that pink eraser of yours. Yeah baby, come for me, I want to hear you moan.'

I see something like lights exploding in my brain and all of a sudden I have such a violent orgasm that I scream. My entire body shudders as I climax again and yet again. My legs are shaking and finally I feel shivers running throughout my body.

'I'm shaking. Thank you.' I deliberately type the words slowly and log off.

sex
with another woman

Introduction

Whether you are gay, straight or in between, fantasizing about someone of the same gender is natural and normal. Sometimes the woman pretends to be a man, sometimes the lovemaking is one-on-one, and sometimes (see the ménage a trois fantasies in Chapter 6) there's a bloke in the mix.

None of this has anything to do with suppressed lesbian urges. If you're straight, your fantasies do not make you gay (ditto if you're gay – if you fantasize about someone of the opposite gender, it doesn't mean you're straight). Studies report that most women will say it's sexy to them to watch another woman's body or think of sexually caressing another woman.

Women are much more likely than men to have same-sex fantasies. On the most basic level, fantasizing about making love with another woman is about variety – something that is totally novel sexually. Sometimes it reflects that your sex partner isn't giving you the type of sex you most desire, especially if the fantasy woman's style is drastically different from his. In these cases, your fantasy woman is an extension of you –

53

THIS is how you would make love to yourself. Perhaps your lover is rough and ready, while you're longing for a lover with a gentle touch.

But these types of fantasies are also a wonderful expression of the joy and acceptance you have of your body, your womanliness, your own sexuality – you can almost say you're embracing yourself.

Patti, 26, PA

My friend Catherine recently admitted to me one night, after having a lot to drink, that she's never had an orgasm. I was a little stunned since she and husband seem to be the perfect couple. But ever since she told me, I have this fantasy where Catherine stumbles in on me masturbating. She whispers, 'Can I join you?' I answer by pulling her close and kissing her deeply. She resists a little, but I can tell she's already a little aroused. Her mouth feels hot. I start rubbing her pussy, my thumb searching out her clitoris. I know I've found her hot spot when she stiffens and moans. She pushes hard against my hand, wanting more. I slide my head between her legs, pushing my tongue in, tasting her. I use my hands to pull her wide apart, my tongue licking her clitoris furiously. I can feel her build and build and then she collapses against me, crying. After a few minutes, she starts caressing my breasts. I tell her not to bother, that I came when she came. Then I massage her clitoris some more, building her up so that when she goes home to her husband, she'll be primed to come.

Helen, 29, massage therapist

Most of the time I think about a summer with my cousin Margaret. Growing up on the Scottish coast was always a nice experience for me. The air smelled of pine trees and the closeness of the sea brought relief from the warm summer temperatures that seemed to make your clothes stick to your skin even after a bath.

Margaret and I grew up together, although she was $3^1/_2$ years older, we were like sisters. We shared everything, even our clothes, until she started blossoming before me. It was late summer, a typical hot, dry day, I decided to go to Margaret's farm to spend the day with her. I had just turned 14 a week earlier and Margaret was going to be 18 in the fall.

That day I wore a red and white checked dress, loose and airy down to my knees, I remember it was comfortable and cool, and a pink ribbon that my Grammy had put in my hair. 'Do not lose it now ... it was your great-grammy's,' I can still hear her say.

Margaret had a way with me ... she would take my hand as we walked along the creek and it seemed so natural ... I didn't know it then, but she was coming on to me.

We eventually ended up at the barn, an imposing structure, as her father was one of the more successful farmers in the area. As we entered the cool darkness of the interior, it surrounded me.

We decided to go up to the loft. The upper structure of the barn is always warmer ... but the hay was fresh and it smelled so sweet. Margaret went up the ladder first and by the time I got up, she was on her hands and knees at the hay-loft door. She was looking for her brothers in the fields.

Her dress was much like mine, loose and breezy. I remember looking at her figure under the light fabric and yearning for the day that I had hips like hers that could hold up my jeans.

She turned over and fell into the hay, a big smile on her face, and she had such a lovely face. Oval with almond-shaped blue eyes and golden hair to her shoulders. Grammy always said 'Golden haired girls are early to bloom,' and that was Margaret. I lay next to her, thinking of how fast the summer was going and how Margaret would be off to university soon.

She must have been thinking the same thoughts. Getting up on one elbow, she brought her face close to mine and looked very intently into my eyes. I had never seen her so serious. It sort of worried me.

'Will you miss me when I'm gone?' she whispered.

My heart ached to tell her how much, but I couldn't. 'Oh yes!' was all I could say.

We lay there looking up at the rafters.

I undid the top two buttons of my dress. I wore no bra – I didn't need one yet – and let the air waft across my tiny breasts, bringing a moment of cool comfort. A drop of sweat trickled between my breasts. Margaret leaned over to me, but her hair fell over her face onto my breasts so I couldn't see what she was doing. I felt her lips touch my breasts and lick off the drop of sweat. It sent a shudder through me.

She lifted her head and brushed that golden hair of hers back from her face to reveal a strange look. Her eyes were glazed over and she had that smile again. The moment stretched on like time had stopped, but the next few minutes are etched in my mind like it happened yesterday.

Margaret reached under my dress to put her hand on my thigh. She lifted my dress over my hips to expose my cotton panties. I was both ashamed and exhilarated. Margaret put her fingers under the elastic band around my upper thigh and pulled aside the fabric. Leaning over, she placed her lips onto the flesh next to my mound and kissed me again. It sent another electric shock through me that almost made me bolt upright. But before I could protest, she had her head down and was kissing a very sensitive spot on the inside of my knee. A 14-year-old girl has no way of knowing there are spots like that on her young body and it was breathtaking. As she proceeded up the inside of my thigh I began to notice the rough texture of her tongue dragging up the soft tissue of my thigh.

Without even feeling her doing it, she had my panties pulled down to my knees and was lifting my legs up to bend them so she could have more comfortable access to my split. She smiled at me again, then lowered her head onto my clitoris ... the shock of her tongue touching me there ... I must have let out a small scream because she gently shushed me and went back to her pleasure.

I was beginning to feel the rumblings of my first orgasm. It built like a thunderstorm and flooded across me like a tidal wave. Time was suspended. When I regained my perception, I was aware of a whooshing sound like listening to seashells with both ears. Slowly, the barn came into focus again. Margaret had her head resting on my shoulder, kissing me softly and stroking my hair. My heart was pounding so loud I thought everyone in town could hear it.

I looked over at Margaret. Her face was glistening all around her mouth with my 'wetness' and she was licking her upper lip. My mind was going in a million different directions. Did she really like 'my taste'? Before I could ask, she reached out and drew me to her. I rolled over onto her and found myself hovering above her groin. I pulled down her panties and was astonished to see she had a shaved mound ... completely hairless. And the aroma – clean and sweet but with an earthy smell that mingled with the animal smells in the barn and the sweet smell of the hay.

I went down to her slit with no shame and tasted the wetness of her body. I found it was like licking honey off a spoon. I'll never forget that first taste as long as I live. And she let out the moan this time. Like an animal, primitive and deep from inside her chest. I worked till I felt the climax building to a peak. As she came, she gushed into my mouth and down my chin. I drank deep.

Time was suspended again. We lay in each other's arms for what seemed like hours.

As the summer wore on, we met at the barn frequently. Margaret went off to school that fall. We eventually lost touch with each other, but I will never forget her – or that summer.

Katie, 22, nanny

Lots of my fantasies include myself with another woman. I used to fantasize only about men. I liked to watch sexy films and often thought about how to please my man. Now I am into my own pleasure.

This is a regular with me: I am with my friend Anne. We have been drinking and we're both feeling randy. We begin kissing. I start roaming over her body. A lick here, a kiss there, a little puff of wind on her cunt. I draw my tongue softly over her love triangle, then push in hard. She moans and thrashes back and forth. I push three fingers deep into her vagina, driving them in and out, extending her orgasm. Anne goes wild, bucking back against my hand. I can feel the juices pouring out of her. I lay back, fingering myself. Anne reaches over and pinches my nipple before burying her head between my thighs. I orgasm in seconds and we collapse in each other's arms.

Stephanie, 26, customer services operator

My friend Maria and I try and have lunch or dinner at least a couple of times a month. We used to work together a few years ago, and we've always enjoyed each other's company. She left to take a slightly better job, and we really have tried to stay in touch. My motives for this though are less than pure. I'm attracted to her. Easy to say, quietly, when nobody can hear me. Impossible to say out loud, especially to her. She's married too. So for now, I simply console myself with lust-filled fantasies about her late at night. During lunch and dinner, I try very hard not to show any signs of attraction – mainly because I've never had a hint of the same feelings from her. All it would take is one definite sign and I'd pounce. At least, I think I would.

Vanessa, 31, teacher

I'd just come out of a serious relationship and needed to just hang out with my best friend. We got really drunk and at one point, she said, 'I really want to kiss you.'

I'd had fantasies about making love to a woman, but never really wanted to go through with it. So I just laughed her off and said she was so pissed that even a woman looked good. But now, what could have happened has become one of my favourite fantasies.

We are about two inches away and I lean in and ever so softly kiss her on the lips. Warm, dry lipstick on lipstick; soft wet tongues touching for the first time. 'Let's go back to my place,' she murmurs.

We get into the car and begin making out. It's a shock to hear your best friend groan with desire, an even bigger shock to feel the hardness of her nipples and discover what sexy lingerie she is wearing. What makes me want to jump to the stars above with sheer delight is easing my hand up her thigh, touching her lacy underwear and then discovering the neat, soft, wetter-than-I-have-ever-known pussy that my fingers dive straight into. Feeling the pleasure rising from her core and hearing it come from her lips onto my neck as I tease her clit and fuck her. The thought 'I'm fucking my best friend and it's great' rises and falls in my consciousness as we bring each other to orgasm after orgasm.

Anonymous

This is a fantasy I have about two women. I don't know who the women are, I just made them up. They are touching each other and getting turned on. I masturbate and time my orgasm to theirs. They come at the same time.

Janice, 30, psychologist

I saw you again today ... I was looking out of my window, out to the rain swept street below. You were sitting in the cafe, next to the window, and I could see your delicate hands wrapped around your cup, steam from the coffee wafting up to your luscious lips. Your skirt was high up on your sexy thighs, your long legs stretched out under the table. I longed to be next to you, to whisper in your ear, to lick your soft earlobes, to taste the sweetness of your lips.

Now, as I lay here, heat rising between my legs, I wonder what it would be like to make love to you. Your breasts must be incredible – I could see their outline under your white shirt. I imagine fondling them, caressing them with my warm hands. As I fantasize, I slip my blouse over my head, baring my own breasts. I slowly start to touch my nipples, making circles with my fingertips, feeling them harden and grow aroused. I imagine that I am rubbing them against your soft skin, pressing them against your breasts. I push down my pants, and slide my panties off, feeling the cool air wash over my hot, naked body. I slide my hands over my belly, and touch my mound, feeling my clit become swollen and excited at the thought of you. My finger finds its way into my slippery cunt hole, pushing inside to feel my wetness. I pretend that I am feeling your cunt, your fragrant wetness is all over my finger. I get two of my fingers all wet, and bring them up to my lips. I suck the juice off my fingers, pretending it is yours, and lick off every drop.

I am getting more aroused, and spread my thighs farther apart. I reach down, with one hand spreading my labia lips open, the other hand exploring the centre of my passion. I rub my clit faster, and feel my own juice pouring out of my pussy, making the satin sheets all wet. I want my fingers to be your fingers – I want to feel your fingers all over my cunt, sliding in and out, pleasuring me. I wish you would lick me with your hot tongue, and lap up my sweet nectar. I am moaning and rolling around the bed, waves of ecstasy washing over me. I sit up and reach over to my nightstand, picking up my vibrator. I lie down again and place the vibrating rod against my clit, rubbing it and spreading my wetness on it. In a burst of passion, I push my dildo into my wide open cunt, and fuck myself with it, shoving it in and out. I am wild with lust, crying out, wanting you to be there to jab your fingers into my cunt and fuck me, make me come, make me spread my juices all over your hand. I squeeze my nipples hard, wanting it to be your mouth sucking and biting them. I remove the vibrator and with my own fingers I stroke my burning clit, faster, faster, until I am gasping for air and screaming out wildly, then in one wild, crazy rush I am coming, calling out for you, moaning and bucking like a wild animal.

I lay there panting, my cum all over my hand and thighs and bed sheets, shivering from a luscious orgasm, and roll over, waiting. I am waiting for you to come home to my loving arms, and my bed.

Lauren, 24, secretary

Being with another woman is a big thing with me. I can't understand why as I wouldn't want to be with one for real. But I love the thought of caressing another woman's breasts and vagina and being with someone who really understands my hot spots.

I've had this fantasy since I was 15. I am with a woman who is unconscious. I am trying to revive her when I notice her shirt is undone. Reaching my hand in, I gently touch the warm top

SEX FANTASIES BY WOMEN FOR WOMEN

of one breast and rub in circles down to her nipple. I am aroused. I can't help it. What I am doing is so exciting.

I put my other hand on my own breast. As I touch the woman, I touch myself. I lean over and take a nipple in my mouth. I gently suck and am delighted when it turns hard. With my knees on the floor and kneeling over the woman, I suck one nipple then the other. I pull on my own nipples with my hands. I am so horny. My underwear is soaked. I move my right hand down and unfasten my own jeans and slip my hand in (this is happening in reality as well as I masturbate myself). I slip my middle finger directly into myself and lift my mouth from the woman's soft flesh long enough to moan.

With my left hand I pull up the woman's skirt and give a small gasp of delight when I see no underwear, just the thick mat of blond pubic hair protecting her spot. I replace my left hand on my own breast and lick my way down to the junction of her legs. I smell the soft warmth and tentatively part the top of the sweet lips with my tongue.

My right hand begins to move faster as a rush of excitement races through my body making my hips rock. I work my tongue down to her opening and thrust it in as far as I can. She moans and I quicken the pace of my thrusts. I thrust into myself with two fingers at the same pace as my tongue, rocking my hips to meet my fingers. I pull harder on my left nipple and rub my breast hard with my palm.

I can feel my muscles tighten. I know I am going to come. I open my mouth as wide as I can and push hard on the woman's core. As my tongue slides in long strokes, the woman's body shudders. She gasps and sighs. We have both come. I quietly leave.

Kelly, 26, PA

I seldom have fantasies during sexual relations – I think. I'm not very inhibited so if I think of something I'd like the man to do or for me to do to him, I usually let him know. It's when I masturbate that I really let my imagination fly.

This is a story I've made up about a friend of mine who I think is really sexy. I know she has been with women and would be with me in a second if I ever showed interest. But I am in a happy straight relationship and would freak out if anything really happened.

We are at my house sitting close together on the couch. The only light is from the TV. You look at me and I turn to you. We kiss a soft, slow, sensual, caring kiss and come apart. We look deeply into each other's eyes and kiss again, this time deeper, fuller and with more intensity pressing to get closer to each other. You kiss my mouth, eyelids, ears, neck, I reciprocate and follow down the curve of your neck. You smell so good. I stop and lead you to my bedroom.

I bend over and light a candle setting a nice glow of light in the room and a faint aroma of peaches. There you are next to my bed, waiting ... I cradle you gently around the waist as we stand at the side of my bed. I'm a bit nervous, because this has been such a long time coming. I can sense your anticipation and wanting without either of us speaking.

I brush a strand of your hair behind your ear and kiss your lips ever so softly and gently as I hold the back of your head. What lips. I love kissing you, taking all of you in. With the other hand, I feel for your breast, cupping it with the palm of my hand (a perfect fit!). I knead it gently as you reach for mine.

We fall onto the bed on top of each other and laugh. You feel the pressure of my body upon yours and we both stop our mirth and get almost serious. There is a connection between us. We both can feel it. You start unbuttoning my shirt and I reach up to unbutton yours. We take each other's off and cast them over the side of the bed and onto the floor. Now we are both in our sports bras.

Your skin feels so good. We caress each other's muscles and outline the definition with our fingertips. I name some of yours and identify them with a kiss. You have such a magnificent body. We sit up to remove our bras. There is no rush here. We are going to take it slow and enjoy the experience for as long as we can. Feeling and exploring every sensation. Making it last.

We are sitting and I touch your breast softly with my hand. We hug and then we touch and hold each other's breasts. Touching from the outside, slowly closing in on the nipple. Circling around and around as we both become very wet and aroused.

You can't wait any longer so you go for my breast with your mouth and take the nipple between your teeth. You suck slowly and lick and massage. I pull you close with a gentle pressure on the back of your head. You look up and give me a devious smile as you nip and suck and lick. You stop and gently kiss my nipple as you go for my other breast and repeat the same routine. Your nipples become pink and erect. We take a break and kiss again and again. Tongues searching each other's teeth and mouths and lips. Now it's my turn. I oblige with a similar routine on each of your breasts. I explore your abdomen with my hand. I push you gently back against my pillows and lay on top of you kissing you deep and long, feeling your breasts against me.

Your breath is quickening. I want to feel you. I kiss your neck, breasts, abdomen, and sides, finding a spot that makes you shiver. A magic spot on your side that excites you. I reach for the fly on your jeans and start to unbutton and unzip you. You catch me off guard and roll me over onto my back and pin my arms as you kiss me with more urgency. You finally let go and start licking and kissing my chest and abdomen, blowing softly as you travel down between my breasts to my navel, underneath my knickers and let your hand rest.

We stop and take off our jeans and underwear. You are so beautiful. Your body is magnificent. So firm and tight and ripe. I could lay next to you like this all day, just staring and marvelling at your beauty. You enjoy the care that I take in my body too. You push me back and climb on top of me, sitting, looking down at me. I want to feel you so bad. You lay down on top of me and put your knee between my legs, searching for my mouth.

Kisses that are hungry, starved, desperate now. A little rougher and more coarse. Face, lips, neck, breathing in my ears, shoulders, breasts, nipples, abdomen, teasing, kneading, licking, nipping. Your other hand slips to the top of my thighs, and I gladly part my legs. I am so wet and I feel your wetness upon me too. You stop and slip down looking up at me with a grin and teasing eyes, kissing and licking here and there as you go. At my thighs, you begin with slow kisses on the inside, a very sensitive spot for me. I can feel your breath on my clitoris as you go from inner thigh to inner thigh. You continue on my thighs and on my legs and behind my knees (another sensitive spot).

A gentle kiss on my clitoris and then you dive in with an urgent hunger, sucking, licking and teasing. I am holding one of your hands and playing with your hair with my other hand. I rock with your rhythm and my breathing speeds up as my sensitivity heightens.

'Stop. Slow down. I want this to last a little longer,' I say and you oblige and the pace decreases. You continue to work me up to almost the point of climax.

'That is so good. Oh! G-d, I'm almost there. I want to feel you inside of me now. Don't stop,' I plead with you as I spread my knees to welcome your fingers inside with a nice rhythm all the way in and almost all the way out. We are in sync with each other, moving and grinding. 'Oh G-d!!!' I'm coming and crashing and falling and it feels so good and I don't want it to stop and I can hardly stand to have it go on. I can hardly breathe, I may have stopped breathing. My heart is pounding.

'OK. Please stop now. That was ... Wow!' You stop your frenzied pace and slow down licking and kissing softly my swollen clitoris, your fingers still wiggling inside of me.

Magda, 29, solicitor

I am single and it is very difficult to find a good lover. I appreciate sex. I need it like bread and butter, sleep, etc. I don't fantasize during sex as a rule. However, if I have a partner who I'm not enjoying, I'll think of this: I am on a train, heading I don't know where – work probably. I immediately notice her when she gets on the train. She has long, dark hair and a perfect hourglass figure. When she sits down next to me, I feel my crotch growing very warm. I'm feeling incredibly sexy in my ruby silk shirt. I'm not wearing a bra and the feel of silk against my nipples is driving me wild. I'm not wearing anything under my wrap-around skirt and flash her as I cross my legs.

She notices, smiles and says, 'Hi.' Her voice is low and sexy. She spreads her legs slightly so that her leg touches mine. It's all I can do not to jump. She leans forward to rummage in her bag, her hair falling over her shoulders. Suddenly, she brings her right hand up and places it so that it touches my thigh and gently moves part of my skirt up a little more.

It all seems so innocent, but I know it's anything but. She reaches deeper into her bag with her left hand, turning her body slightly towards me. As she does, I see that her left breast is completely exposed. All I want is to reach across and stroke her nipple.

She finally finds and removes a book from her bag. She begins reading, her body slightly turns towards me. She moves her right hand and brushes her lovely hair back from her face, and as she does, her elbow gently brushes my left breast. I can barely stand it!

I look around. The car is empty and I decide to play along. I turn slightly towards her, and feign an interest in her book. I place my left elbow on the back of the seat just behind her head, and prop my head in my hand. 'What is it that you are reading?' I ask, looking directly at her. She turns and meets my gaze, and says, 'A story about two women who meet on a train and have a sexual encounter.' 'Just one?' I ask, turning slightly more towards her so that my skirt opens more, revealing the creamy inside of my thighs.

As I look up again at her, she's glancing down at my thighs, and ever so slightly moves her hips forward. She laughs quietly and drops the book back in her bag. Then she places her hand on the inside of my thigh. I move my legs further apart, and my skirt splits to reveal my mound. Her hand moves up even slightly more, stopping just short of my lips. I can feel how wet my cunt is getting. I sweep away a few stray hairs from her face, then stroke that softness of her sweet skin. She closes her eyes, and moves her mouth to kiss my hand. At first, her open lips gently stroke my fingers, then her tongue lightly caresses my palm as I hold it open to her. She takes my first three fingers into her mouth completely, swirling her tongue around and over them, sucking on them deeply, looking directly into my eyes.

My clit is throbbing and aching. As if on cue, her right hand moves to gently brush against my pubic hair, and then my lips. I felt my breath catch in my throat, and close my eyes. She takes my hand and presses it against her breast. I take the hint and gently squeeze her boob. Now it's her turn to gasp. I move my hand to the underside of her full breast and let my thumb gently flick her tit. Each flick of that huge, hard nipple creates a throb in my own clit.

After a quick glance – the car is still miraculously empty – I lick her breast, and then suck it deeply into my mouth. She moves her hand into my lips, up to my clit. Oh, God! I think I'll explode. Her fingers are working so quickly and lightly, and I can tell mine is not the first cunt that she has explored.

Her left hand holds my head in place, and I keep working my mouth against her breast; licking, sucking and biting. I move my hand under her skirt. She parts her legs even more and I feel her wet, pulsating pussy. My fingers go inside her without a problem. She thrusts her hips upward toward my hand, and I start fucking her. She pulls her skirt up over her cunt and up to her waist. My mouth never leaves her breast except to look down at my fingers pumping in and out of her cunt, wet and sticky.

Her hand is still moving, with what seems like the speed of light, over my clit. I feel that any minute I'll scream with orgasm, but I keep myself at bay and move my legs even further apart, so she has easier access to my wet, swollen pussy. As she slides her fingers into my hole, with her palm still rubbing my hard little clit, I start pumping my own hips, both to fuck her fingers and to rub my clit against her hand.

She comes. Loudly. A few moments later, so do I. As we straighten our clothing, the train pulls into the next station. People swarm on. She slips out, giving me a wink as she exits.

Paula, 24, painter

My fantasy starts in the middle. I am naked with another woman. I can't clearly see her face. She is nibbling at my neck while we press our cunts into each other's thighs. Her mouth finds mine and we kiss long and deep, tongues swirling.

She pulls away and takes my hand, leading me to the bedroom. She directs me to lie down on the bed.

'Now, my sweet, I'm going to suck and tease your pussy until you beg me to stop,' she says. 'And I'm not stopping at just one. You'll come at least twice, or more. Please, make yourself comfortable.'

With that said, she kisses my mouth, then each breast and nipple, then my stomach, my navel, my mound of hair, and locks her mouth right over my clit. She sucks it like a baby sucks a bottle, her lips pursed and mouth moving.

Oh, the splendour of it all! What a perfect moment! For the next hour, she sucks my clit, and fucks me with her hands, both in my cunt and in my ass, sometimes fucking both holes and licking me all at once.

And climax I do! My first orgasm is explosive, and then the next beyond anything I've ever experienced. The third makes me almost lose consciousness. She keeps her promise.

I have versions of this fantasy once or twice a week.

Anonymous

I am naked.

Standing on a gentle slope somewhere, hot soft wind brushes against my body. A soft glow comes from a small light just in front of me, while behind is complete darkness. I step forward, following the light. As I reach the light, I see another one, slightly farther away, leading down the slope. As I follow the soft lights, I think about what awaits me at the end.

Reaching the bottom of the slope, I see a covered platform with a bed on it. I step onto the platform, and light bathes my body. A woman steps from the shadows, also nude. She approaches me slowly, her hands reaching out for me. Her soft hands brush the side of my neck sliding over my shoulders. Her hands cup my breasts, fingers playing with my hardening nipples.

She kisses me, her lips pressing gently against mine. Her mouth slides over my skin, tongue exploring me completely. She kneels between my legs, spreading them. Her mouth covers my pussy, sucking my clit gently into her mouth. Her hands pull me harder against her mouth as her tongue probes deeply within me. A greased finger slides slowly into my anus, slowly pumping in and out of me.

I close my eyes as an orgasm quickly approaches. A second finger joins the first in my asshole, the pace picking up slightly. A flood of come is released from me, covering her face. I open my eyes to look at her face covered in my juices, but the woman has gone.

Linda, 39, accountant

I have had a few experiences with women. This fantasy is from a flirtation I had with a girl who lived in my college dorm. We shared a shower room with four other women. One evening, we both wanted to take a shower at the same time. We joked about taking one together, but decided that she would go first in the end. This is my fantasy about what could have happened.

I tell Samantha to go ahead and use the shower first. She smiles and suggests I join her.

She turns on the shower and steps in, pulling me behind her.

The water is warm, with good water pressure. Samantha unwraps a bar of soap and begins to lather it up in her hands. She pulls me away from the jet and begins to soap my entire body. Her hands slide over and under my breasts, my arms, my neck, and then my lower body. When her hands slide between my legs with the soap, I feel a rush of arousal go through me.

I lean against one side of the shower while she soaps my back and my bottom, one finger sliding into my bum as it goes past. I moan as she kneels on the floor, soaping my legs, hands once again sliding back to my cunt. She pushes me under the shower, letting the warm pulsing water remove the soap from my body.

As the last remnants of the soap are washing from my body, her hands explore me firmly. She hands the soap to me. She steps back from the stream of water and I begin rubbing the soap all over her body. When I reach between her legs, I rub the soap across her lips. My fingers spread her open and the soap now strokes her clit.

Her legs weaken a little and she holds onto me for balance. My arms grab her and pull her tight against me, my fingers stroking her bottom. I manage to slide one finger deep within her backside. Our mouths meet as I pull her back under the stream of water with me, washing off the soap. My fingers slide down between her legs to stroke her clit. She comes again.

By now the water has begun to cool off a little, so we leave the shower, towelling each other dry. We dress quickly and head back to our respective rooms.

Louisa, 26, model

I have fantasies of sucking voluptuous girls' tits and touching their round bellies and hugging them. Usually I try to think of someone I know – an acquaintance or friend or someone I've noticed. I have fantasies of rubbing up against them.

Simone, 25, travel agent

My daydreaming fantasies usually end up in masturbation. I must have had other daydreaming fantasies, as I have been masturbating since I was about 11, but I can't seem to remember any except this one. I pretend I am a man making love to a beautiful woman. I am gentle and considerate and make sure she has a climax. Then I come. She loves me for being so caring of her and licks me from head to toe. By the end, I have turned back into a woman and we go off and live together.

Tracy, 20, student

My best mate and I are hanging out as usual, lounging around on a Sunday morning after a night of watching *Dawson's Creek* on my bed. This is something we actually do. But in my fantasy, she turns to me to say something and suddenly our eyes lock. Stomachs turning, we both close our eyes and lean towards each other. Then, before either of us can even say anything, we are making love.

Beth, 24, researcher

I have always had lesbian fantasies, although I have never had a lesbian experience. This is one of my favourites. I am on a business trip with my boss. She is an attractive redhead and I think she may be into women. Anyway, we are sharing a hotel room.

We have had a very successful trip and picked up some lucrative new business. All night, during our celebratory dinner, the sparks have been flying. We order champagne and get a little giddy.

When we get back to our room, as soon as the door was shut, Anna takes me into her arms, kissing me softly on the lips. Her fingers trace paths up and down my body, touching some of my more sensitive spots. Her tongue traces a trail up the inside of my arm, turning and flicking the wrist once again. A moan springs from my lips as she turns me around and begins licking the back of my neck, then down between my shoulder blades. I can feel her mouth travelling down my body, exploring my buttocks. Her tongue flicks against my bum, probing inside it, pressing deep within.

She pushes me gently down on the bed, my hard nipples rubbing against the cover. I look back and see her removing her clothes. I felt her soft breasts press against my back as she moves on top of me, teeth pulling gently at my ear. Her fingers slide underneath me, pressing into my vagina, pulling me hard against her. I can feel her moist hot cunt pressing against my backside.

She begins to move slowly down my body, her mouth exploring every part of me as she works her way downwards. Her tongue finds a new spot and flicks out, pressing against my skin. She moves past my pussy, trailing her tongue down my legs, the backs of my knees, then down around my ankles.

I turn over and pull her up against me, our breasts pressing together, our cunts pushing hard to meet. I slide my hand between us, feeling both sets of lips pressing against my hand.

We writhe in ecstasy and come over and over, collapsing in each other's arms for the night. The next morning, on the train back to town, we pretend nothing has happened ... until the next business trip.

Belinda, 27, investment banker

I've had fantasies about sleeping with another woman. We're alone together having a drink and we start talking about sex. We get really horny and, since there aren't any men around, we start exploring each other. We don't kiss much, but we massage each other's bodies. We end up having oral sex and I have the most explosive orgasm ever.

Do I want this fantasy to become a reality? I can't say I wouldn't want to have sex with another woman, although I think I'm too inhibited to ever try it. I'm not a lesbian or bisexual and wouldn't want to have relationships with women, but an experimental session with a woman I'd never see again would be the ideal situation. I like the idea of someone knowing exactly what turns you on because they have the same body and know how it works. Even with private lessons, I'm sure a bloke couldn't be as good at oral sex as a woman!

Sometimes my fantasy involves my partner and another woman so I get the best of both worlds.

forced
fantasies

Introduction

No! No! Yes!

Being forced to have sex against your will is – surprisingly – the most common erotic daydream there is for women. In fact, rape fantasies are far more common than rapes themselves. Studies have found that 51 per cent of women have fantasized about being forced to have sex, while a third imagined: 'I'm a slave who must obey a man's every wish.'

Basically, these fantasies are NOT about being raped but about being overpowered sexually. Women who find submission fantasies sexually arousing are very clear that they have no wish to be raped in reality.

There is a huge difference. In their fantasies, women call the shots and control every aspect of what occurs. So while there's some force involved on the man's part – i.e., a man overpowers a woman against her will – unlike real-life attacks, these fantasies aren't violent or brutal. The man is often a hot hunk whose restraint is simply overwhelmed by the woman's high babe quotient.

These fantasies serve the same psychological purpose as scenes of irresistibility. It's different means to the same end – we want to be desired.

It used to be thought that the rape fantasy was a favourite with women who felt guilty about having sex as a way of giving themselves permission to experience carnal pleasure – being forced cleared them of responsibility for their lust. But it's now known that it's the women who have had MORE sexual experience who are more likely to have forced sex fantasies. This suggests that these women tend to be more open to explore a variety of sexual stimuli – including rape fantasies.

Another possibility – maybe you are powerful in real life and you live to give it all up and totally relinquish control in your fantasies.

Conversely, if you fantasize about forcing someone to have sex with you, then it could mean that you feel like you have no control in your real life so you like to be controlling in your fantasies. Experts say that these fantasies often have to do with how power is dealt with in all of your relationships – if you feel it's unequal, you'll often redress the balance in your daydreams, even your sexual ones.

Then again, it could simply be an attempt to 'experience' the aggressive side of sex.

Venetia, 28, estate agent

A dark, tall man passes me on the street and looks at me passionately. I keep walking. He follows me home and pushes his way into my house. He grabs me. I try to get away. He is breathing hard and so am I. He pulls my legs apart and pushes his penis inside. He is enormous. I fight to get away, but he keeps pushing hard. Against my will, I start to respond. He is filling me in a way I have never been filled before. We both come quickly and violently.

I use this fantasy to spice things up with my lover sometimes, especially when he seems about to come before me.

Maria, 26, computer programmer

I'm fascinated by the idea of domination. In my fantasy, I am with two other women – co-workers. We are in a room with a man who is a client of our company. He is often rude to us – simply, I suspect, because we are women. The three of us pin him to the floor and strip him. He tries to get away but I start sucking his penis until it becomes hard. Then I sit on top of him until I climax. The other two women satisfy themselves in the same way. Then we leave him tied up and unsatisfied.

Lydia, 34, chef

I have had an on-line flirtation for a few months now. We met in a chat room on cooking and somehow our conversation drifted away from the trivial recipe exchanging to the sexual. We started exchanging secrets and facts about ourselves that the other couldn't quite believe. Then he started discussing how it would be if we were together, making love, specifically talking about oral sex. I eagerly gave my opinion, and it appeared that both of us equally liked to give and receive. I quickly discovered how much he wanted to please me, though I didn't share with him that the feeling was mutual. I also found out that he had a raging erection and wasn't planning to do anything about it at the moment. Shame. How I wished I could have.

Towards the end of the conversation, he asked what I would do if he came up to me and asked for a trade. I told him he'd just have to find that out. And the most interesting question he posed was if I was concerned that he might attack me sometime. I told him no, I wasn't concerned; I trusted him.

In my fantasy, that is exactly what happens. The doorbell rings and when I answer it, I know it is him. He doesn't say a word. He just comes in and overpowers me. I want him to stop, but at the same time, what he is doing to my body feels so good, that I hope he doesn't.

Finally, just as he is about to enter me, I groan. He laughs and teases me by hovering above my opening. Frustrated, I grab him and pull him into me. He laughs again as I come, knowing he has won me over.

After I have come, he leaves without saying a word.

Olivia, 24, trainee accountant

The doorbell rings. A stranger is there. He overpowers me and says, 'You must do as I say.'

Scared, I nod.

'Spread your legs apart so that they touch each wall of this hallway.'

I do so and he lifts my skirt and slides underneath me to lick my pussy. I try not to respond, but it feels so good. He begins lapping up my juices, slower and then faster, as I come all over his face.

He laughs and leaves.

Naomi, 24, librarian

When I've got a boyfriend, my fantasies are usually about him rather than a stranger. Sometimes during sex, when he's going down on me, I'll focus on some scenario to help me orgasm. They're things I'd actually like to do at some point and they're pretty tame really.

I like the idea of being at a party and him dragging me into the loo while there are people waiting outside in a queue. He's absolutely bursting to have sex with me and he bends me over the bath and takes me from behind. It's the fact that he has to have me NOW that turns me on. Also the ways he's being so forceful about it is really exciting. I like the feeling of being dominated.

My other party sex scene is him forcing me to have sex on top of the coats even though we know someone might come in. Someone does come in – a friend of his – and my boyfriend tells him to stay and look at my body and see how horny I am. His mate wants to have sex with me and even though I say no, my boyfriend tells him to go ahead. We all end up in a mad lovely tangle on the bed. Then it all fades away.

Rachel, 32, medical sales rep

I have this fantasy whenever I masturbate. It is based on a real experience I had with my boyfriend. He is the best lover ever.

My boyfriend and I are making love. His fingers are sliding beneath me, three of them pushing into my cunt, his thumb rubbing my clit. Suddenly he stops.

'Kneel on the bed.'

I do. He comes up behind me, pulls my hands back and ties them. He stands next to me stroking his penis.

'Do you want it?' he whispers. 'Do you want me to fuck you?'

'Yes, do it,' I whisper back.

As he goes behind me, he says only one word: 'Watch.' I know exactly what he means. There is a mirror on the dresser that gives a good view of the bed. I turn my head and watch him slide his penis into my pussy. He grabs my hips and pulls me back against him, my wrists squeezed between us. He continues to fuck me slowly, occasionally pulling his penis out and sliding it up the crack of my ass.

He pulls out and, giving me a wicked smile, displays a large dildo. He spreads lubricant over the head.

'It's too big,' I protest.

'Let's try it,' he coaxes.

The head presses slowly against my anus. I press back against it and feel the head slide past my sphincter. I can't believe it is going in so easily. I watch in the mirror as it slides deep into my ass. He begins to pump the dildo in and out while he fucks my cunt. His free hand slides over my body, caressing me.

I am whimpering, but with pleasure. I come, but my boyfriend keeps up the pumping until I have come again and again until I lose count and collapse.

I have this fantasy occasionally – it overlaps into masturbation usually. It has never actually happened, although I think I would like to experience it – but only with my boyfriend.

Christina, 31, scientist

I've always wanted a women to take charge of me and my husband and have her way with us. I fantasize that she makes me lick her clit while my husband is inside her, and she makes me lick his balls while he is fucking her. And when it slips out, she makes me put it back in with my mouth. After she has had many orgasms, she sits back and sips a glass of wine or cognac while she makes us suck each other off. Then she has her way with us again.

Margaret, 34, housewife

I have found that many women have several different forms of 'rape fantasies'. I know I do. Women obviously do not want the extreme violence of an actual rape, but often, they do like the element of surprise, and the submissive behaviour that these fantasies allow you to have. To tell my husband 'no' as we role-play, and to have him 'force' me, gives me a sense of his desire and want for me. It arouses me very much. But this does not mean that I want to be raped.

Karen, 24, PA

I fantasize about being taken – a beautiful stranger overcoming me against my will, stripping me down and making forceful love to me. I don't want it, but I also don't want him to stop. I think I am seeking out this sense of belonging. I want to know I am HIS, and he wants me totally, desires me fully, and possibly even demands (in a very loving way).

Linda, 21, student

Don't ask me why I want a rape fantasy. It boggles my mind. I was raped when I was 15. The violation was approximately four hours, and I still have the scars to show it. I was grabbed by my hair and yanked down my back porch (concrete), on my back, so that is the one I will live with forever. Thank God I can't see the scratch marks.

However, I know, after therapy, that what I experienced was not sex. It was a young man tortured by his step-father, and after a severe beating he came to my house and I comforted him. He knew he could overpower me and he did.

My ravishment fantasy is something completely different to me than rape. For me, it is sex that is still playful. I don't know if I am searching this activity out to help me play back the past or what. But this is more of what I am wanting. I won't be graphic because not everyone wants to hear this sort of thing.

But this is more of my fantasy ... maybe some would see it as ravishment.

It would take place in a very scary place ... a cemetery, or slaughter-house, or something of that nature. He would be a 'first-date'. It would combine the element of surprise with the ultimate fear. It would be sexual, not abusive. Very seductive, very naughty. But I want him to terrorize me. I don't want to know what is coming next.

I would love to be tied up in the middle of the room ... helpless ... while he tortures, and taunts, and teases me.

Does this make sense? Perhaps it is ravishment, but it is in the utmost severe meaning of the word.

Linda, 30, police officer

I would love to be with a woman and another guy. The man has to be there, but I would love it if he made me do things with the girl, like suck her to make her wet for him. Then I would have to eat his cum out of her pussy after he came inside of her. I lick her ass and tongue it too. Then I suck and swallow his dick and cum so she can just sit back and masturbate while watching.

The point is they could make me do absolutely anything.

Anne, 28, radio technician

This is my fantasy, and it's based on something true. This guy was the biggest asshole – an alcoholic and a womaniser – but I was with him for a very long time. He never had anything to say, but he had such a big dick, I always dreamed about him. The best was the one where I hear a knock at the door. I open it. He is out of breath. He pants, 'I've been watching you for a long time' and pushes me against a wall. We start kissing and what he says is enough to make me wet: 'Do what you want to me.'

This is where my fantasy takes over from the dream. I strip him down and tie his hands and legs together. I light a candle and start dripping wax all over his body, slowly. He is squirming and crying, which is an incredible turn-on because he is such a big masculine guy. I can't believe I can reduce him to this. But at the same time, his penis is rock hard.

I take a feather and drag it all over his body. He wants to come, but I refuse to allow him, reducing the pressure whenever it looks like he's going to lose control. Finally, I can't take it anymore. Still, I am in charge. I climb on top of him (in reality, whenever we made love, I would be on the bottom) and set the pace, making it last for hours, until he is literally crying and begging me. Finally, I let us both come.

Anonymous

My fantasy would be to have long passionate sex on the beach just by the water's edge as the sun is coming up. I would be the one initiating the sex – which is something I normally don't do. I know I would enjoy the experience to the fullest because I would be in charge and I would be deciding when it is time to come (often, my lovers are too quick for me).

Helen, 30, photo researcher

I had this boss, Jack, who was gorgeous. We had a flirtation going. Nothing ever happened, but I fantasized what might have...

He calls me into his office.

'Sit down,' he commands, 'You know I find you very beautiful.'

I ask him if this was why I had been called into the office.

'Why do you think?' answers Jack. He jumps up from behind his desk and stretches his broad body. Not looking at me, Jack takes off his tie and unbuttons his shirt. I stare at him, amazed. He is beautiful, chiselled abs, well-formed pectorals and the smoothest tanned bronze skin. I look into his eyes, deep blue. They are beckoning me to come to him.

'Take something of yours off,' Jack says firmly.

I start to walk out – I need the job too much to risk this. But he tells me to stop or I will get fired.

'Look at my body,' he commands.

Jack takes off his shirt completely. His arms are large and strong, now I can see all of his torso. I begin to feel wet. He takes off his trousers and stands in front of me, his erection squeezed against designer boxer shorts. I get up, against my will, walk towards him and throw myself against his body. I can smell his expensive aftershave, sense the warmth of his body and feel his heart beat. He undresses me, peeling off my blouse, expertly taking away my bra, leaving only my knickers. I half-protest – I am hot but feel like he is forcing me to do something against my will – but he ignores me.

'Fuck, babe, you turn me on,' Jack says, feeling my breasts in his hands, massaging my nipples.

I can't. He pushes down his boxer shorts. His cock is long and thick and throbbing with sexual excitement. He pushes my head down to take it in my mouth and suck hard. He groans loud enough for the office to hear.

Ripping off my knickers he pushes me onto the desk and pushes his hard cock inside me. I can't help myself. I scream in ecstasy. As he pumps faster and faster on top of me, I feel the muscular contours of his body. His face is wild and I feel with every thrust he is closer to orgasm.

I feel everything build up within me, just staring at this perfect body. I let go, the intensity of my orgasm takes us both by surprise. He spurts cum in three slowing thrusts inside me.

Withdrawing and picking up his clothes, he says, 'Thank you, Helen. That will be all.'

I get dressed and return to my desk, sure everyone knows from my flushed face what has gone on.

Amanda, 21, student

I create fantasies not only to bring myself to orgasm, but also to enjoy myself and get lost in the sensual pleasure. In one favourite fantasy, I imagine being on my king-size bed with my hands tied to the headboard. Because of the bondage, I have no control over my husband and the two small, beautiful women who massage me with oil and take turns pleasuring me. They make me come over and over until I am literally spent and sobbing. Then I sleep really well.

Vicky, 31, writer

Today I am his mistress and he is my slave.

'Do you understand fully what this means?' I ask.

'Yes' he replies, only to be reprimanded.

'When you are spoken to you will answer "Yes Mistress" and if you are not spoken to you will not speak at all ... is that very clear?' A very quiet 'yes Mistress' can be heard. I am not sure that he is intrigued by my plan, but decide to proceed.

'I want you to be naked always in my presence, and your sole purpose is for my pleasure. Now if you would undress and run a shower for me,' I demand. He does as he is told and I can now see he is aroused by this new experience.

After he undresses me, I enter the bathroom and hand him my razor. I step into the shower and tell him to shave me. He lathers my legs with shave cream. When my legs are shaved nicely, I tell him that he did a marvellous job, but I want my pussy shaved. His eyes widen but he sets to work carefully shaving me, his fingers sometimes entering me, sometimes spreading me open, but he remains obedient and keeps at his task until it is complete. His cock is very hard now and is jumping in front of him as he follows my next order to wash my body and shampoo my hair. His hands glide over my body, but never linger and I am getting very aroused. The water cascades over my body as I tell him to enter the shower and kneel before me.

'I want you to make me cum!' His tongue darts into my hot pussy as he spreads my now clean-shaven lips apart. I feel his slippery fingers toying with my ass and soon one, then two fingers are churning inside it. As he sucks my clit between his teeth, I tense, then scream, as a raging orgasm washes over my body.

I push his face hard against me and cum for what seems like an eternity. My knees buckle but he senses my predicament and steadies me without stopping his attack on my body.

When I compose myself, I tell him to wash himself and then masturbate while I watch. 'Yes Mistress,' he replies happily, glad that release is in sight. He begins to stroke his rock hard cock and in a very short time his body tenses, the muscles in his legs ripple.

I order him to STOP! He looks at me, his eyes pleading, but he does as he is told. We get out of the shower and after he dries me and then himself, we retire to the bedroom.

I tie him to the posts of my brass bed, and gently bend to lick the purple head of his hardness. I tease him, sucking his cock and licking it with my tongue. After a while, I get a vibrator and push it in and out of my pussy until I am on the brink of another orgasm.

I love watching the look on his face as he watches me masturbate. He's straining against his binds.

'Mistress, may I speak?' I nod to him and he begs to be allowed to cum. 'Please Mistress, I am going to die, I am in pain ... let me bring you to another orgasm and then be allowed to cum.'

I smile at his sincerity, but before I set him free I take the now wet vibrator and insert it slowly into his ass. He groans in a mixture of pleasure and pain, then delight spreads across his face.

Finally, I release the silk ties. I take him into my arms, his cock enters me. He is hotter than I can remember him being. He takes me forcefully and soon we orgasm together and then settle into a long session of lovemaking. As the sun rises in the morning sky, we fall asleep cuddled against each other spent and content.

Katrina, 28, restaurant manager

I am a fragile princess chained in a dungeon by an evil monster, an immortal outcast from the underworld. He visits me, sometimes three or four times a day and each time I become aroused in fearful anticipation. He instructs me on which positions to assume and I must obey – or be punished. After he leaves, I rest and eat and wait for him to come again. He is my existence.

Cherine, 29, manager

I agree to let a guy who has recently broken up with me come over. Instead of making the first move – the way things usually happen – I tease him, taking off my clothes, straddling his lap. He tries to take control – he becomes desperate, pleading – but I say no, he can't enter me. After I orgasm, I roll over and fall asleep, leaving him unsatisfied.

Alyssa, 31, merchandiser

I am a successful professional woman, self-confident and self-assured. I demand and receive respect in my relationships; I'm not afraid of making major decisions. To be dominated in my relationships – sexually or otherwise – goes against everything I believe in and yet ... my boyfriend's innuendos about dominance and submission have preyed on my mind constantly. Tim has mentioned several times the idea of my becoming his 'slave' for the weekend, although he quickly laughs it off. My fantasies have become invaded by possibilities. This is one that I am thinking of sharing with Tim.

The phone rings just before my alarm is set to ring. Bringing it to my ear, I hear Tim's voice softly telling me to call in sick and come to his house. He needs me. I impulsively say yes, it is Friday anyway and I have put in a hard week. I hang up the phone. I call my office and tell them I will not be in and head for the shower.

The phone is ringing again as I step from the shower. I grab a towel and run for the phone. Before I can say hello I hear Tim's voice. 'Wear your black trench coat and heels and nothing else.'

The line goes dead.

As I dry my hair I think about what he has said. It is a silly idea ... crazy in fact, and yet, it excites me. My curiosity is piqued and it appeals to the 'wild child' of my youth that I now keep buried within me. He doesn't live that far away ... what can possibly happen from my house to his? And I will never know his plans unless I play the game.

It is a game, isn't it? I take my leather duffel bag and hurriedly pack jeans and a cotton sweater and sneakers to wear later. I put on black heels and then my trench coat. The coat feels cold against my skin as I tie the belt tightly around my waist.

The sun is already shining brightly but the air is still cold as I head out of the door. I can feel the chill under my coat as I walk to my car. It seems to be teasing my thighs and then higher, in stark contrast to the heat I am feeling between my legs.

My body tingles all over as I drive and by the time I reach Tim's house I am so aroused, I can feel my wetness seeping onto my thighs. My hand trembles as I reach for his door.

The door opens just as I touch the knob and instead of finding Tim naked and ready for me as I had expected, he is dressed in my favourite black suit. He leads me through the door and stands back admiring me.

'Open your coat,' he speaks softly yet firmly. I open my coat and stand before him, revealing my naked body.

'Very nice. You have followed my orders well. Take off your coat and listen to my words carefully. Today you are mine ... I adore you and I am going to give you more pleasure than you have ever imagined possible, but you must remember you belong to me. You will do nothing without being told to do it by me. I will make all your decisions for you. I will be your total source of energy and power. Do you understand?'

I can barely speak, my mind is racing so fast but I find my voice and whisper a quiet 'Yes.'

Tim smiles, his eyes warm and caring, then he speaks again: 'I can tell you are very aroused. That pleases me but I must go to the office for an hour or so. I want you to pleasure me before I go. On your knees. Show me how much you like to lick and suck my cock.'

As if under a spell, I am on my knees opening Tim's zipper and releasing his semi-erect penis. I feel him growing harder as my lips caress the head of his cock. I lick the shaft, moving my tongue firmly around its thickness, wetting it so my mouth can move more easily up and down its length. I feel his hands on the back of my head, guiding me and as he increases the speed of my movements I suck harder. My hand drops between my legs and finds my clitoris. As I begin circling it, electricity is coursing through my body.

Again Tim speaks. 'Move your hand away. I didn't tell you could touch yourself, did I? I will tell you what to do.' He moves my head steadily as he speaks. I can feel his body tensing with orgasm as he holds my head firmly against his groin. 'Swallow. We must keep my suit clean so I can go to work.' He groans just before he comes in a swift rush.

Tim steps back and while straightening his clothing, he quietly explains his plans. 'While I am gone, you will remain naked. You are not to touch yourself or find release in anyway. I have prepared the VCR for you. When I am gone you are to sit and watch the video I have selected for you. I should be home by the time it is over, but I want you to know I will be thinking of you while I complete my work.' With that, he closes the door behind him and was gone.

My nakedness leaves me feeling exposed and vulnerable. My thoughts are jumbled and yet I know I find this whole scene incredibly arousing. I also immediately know I will follow his orders and see where they lead me.

I sit on the leather sofa and its cool smooth surface sends a chill through me. I turn on the VCR and wait to see what Tim has picked for me. It is an erotic adventure into a woman's dreams. The photography is superb and each segment brings me closer to the brink of orgasm. I sit mesmerized as a gorgeous Dominatrix is brought to ecstasy by a willing slave woman. While I watch a man licking and sucking this same woman's dripping pussy, I find myself reaching once again for my clit.

Remembering Tim's orders, I move my hand away but I am finding it more difficult to sit still each minute.

Just when the video is ending, the door opens and Tim walks in.

'How are you doing? Did you do as you were told?' he questions. I whisper 'Yes.' 'Then come here,' he orders. 'Did you enjoy the movie? Let me check.' I nod my head as I walk toward him, not trusting my voice. I stand before him and wait for what seems like a very long time.

Tim takes his fingers and enters me gently. His thumb brushes my clit and a moan escapes my lips. He speaks while looking directly into my eyes, 'Ahhh – yes, you have been a very good girl. You are very wet. You will be rewarded.' His thumb continues its magic on my hard clitoris but stops abruptly just as I am nearing orgasm. I start to speak, but Tim brings his wet fingers to my lips to quiet me. 'Shhh! Come to the bedroom and undress me. I want to be more comfortable.'

I undress him slowly. I yearn to kiss him and feel the warmth of his body next to mine but remain focused on the task at hand.

Each button seems to take forever beneath my trembling fingers. Finally Tim gives me permission to touch his body if I so desire. When he is naked my fingers play in his chest hair and my lips tease his nipples. I can feel his hardness reaching toward me, but as I move my hips to place Tim's cock between my legs, he moves away.

He tells me to lie on the bed. He places pillows under my head and makes sure I am comfortable. He drizzles oil onto my nipples and then slowly down my body. Each drop feels hot as my body responds. I lay there not moving, waiting for his touch but it doesn't come. I begin to squirm. After what seems like an eternity, he begins to massage the oil into my waiting body. He starts at my breasts, rolling my nipples between his fingers and kneading my breasts with the palm of his hands. Slowly he massages me, varying the pressure. His fingers are now slippery enough to slip off my nipples when he pinches them and I arch my back to find them again. My hips begin to move in a steady rhythm and my moans are almost constant now. I want Tim more than I have ever wanted anyone before. I feel my sex swollen and ready, but no release is in sight.

He moves his hands down across my belly. Taking one finger he lightly draws little circles in my pubic hair, then reaches in between my wet lips to tease my clit. I at once move against him but he pulls away. He reaches lower to my inner thighs and firmly massages them. He takes his time and moves up again, taking the lips of my pussy between his fingers and stroking each one over and over. He opens my pussy lips and touches the velvet smoothness of their inner lining. He strokes his finger up and down sometimes with a touch so light I can barely feel it.

My body is screaming for release. Every nerve ending seems to be on fire. Every touch of his fingers sends me reeling with a passion I have never known. Tim speaks softly for the first time since he has touched me. 'You must trust me completely. You will not climax until I give you permission.'

He lowers his body between my legs and spreads my legs wide. His fingers open my pussy and he lets me feel his hot breath against my wetness. I try to move up to his mouth but he holds me firmly. I wait and try to focus on work, anything but the intensity of the moment.

His tongue touches my clitoris and I gasp at his touch. He teases it with the tip of his tongue, then begins sucking it gently between his lips. His fingers enter me, spreading me open and bringing me to the edge once again. He waits until I subside. Then, relentlessly, he resumes licking. He stops again ... waiting for me to slow myself down. This time it takes longer. He knows I am reaching my limits. Soon the pleasure of the tension he has created will turn to a painful experience. He will let me build one more time and then grant my release.

He lies at my side caressing my body as my breathing returns to normal. He brings me a drink of water. When I seem to be calmed, he once again moves between my legs. There is no holding me back now. I quickly return to an exaggerated state of arousal. My hips are moving wildly beneath his head. My breath comes in gasps and this time, when Tim feels my body tensing, he sucks my clit between his teeth and pinches my nipples firmly. I scream as my orgasm overtakes me. The spasms are never-ending and my body shakes as Tim very gently sucks my hot nectar into his mouth. The room goes dark for several seconds while my total focus is on wave after wave of delicious orgasm coursing through me.

He moves his body up and guides his cock into me. Slowly he strokes in and out ... his control of himself is as all-consuming as his control of me has been. My hips are moving faster beneath him. Our bodies become one, moving in unison with one goal. Our orgasms come on top of one another ... both of us burning with a fire like none before.

Spent, we lay beside one another ... touching, kissing. I await his next command.

Haley, 29, teacher

I have never tried bondage but have always been curious. This is how I imagine it would go. I am out on a date with a man I have been seeing regularly. We have made love before, but tonight, as he undresses me, he has a mischievous smile on his face. He turns toward the nightstand and pulls something out. He turns back, giving me a questioning look as he holds up a handful of long red silk scarves.

A slight shiver goes down my spine, but I nod slightly.

He indicates I should lie on the bed. I lie down, spreading my arms and legs, my hands grasping the headboard. He slides a scarf around one of my ankles, twisting it and tying it to the footboard. My other leg is soon spread and tied down. He moves up the bed and fastens one wrist to the headboard, then the other one. Finally a scarf is tied firmly over my eyes, obscuring my view.

I hear him get off the bed and exit the room. He returns shortly and sits down beside me. I feel liquid land between my breasts, dribbling down my cleavage.

He teases me for what feels like hours. I am brought almost to orgasm again and again, but he always backs off on his stimulation before I actually come. By now, I am begging him to release me, crying and writhing in a way that I never usually do when I make love.

Suddenly, it's quiet again. I hear him rooting around in a nightstand by the bed. Suddenly, I feel a flick on my skin. He is tapping me with what feels like a leather riding crop. I expect to hate it, but it actually leaves my skin tingling.

'Okay?' whispers my date.

Hesitantly, I nod my head. He flicks again and again. I feel myself coming. Just as I explode, he fills me with his penis and whips us both to a frenzied orgasm.

Wendy, 27, waitress

My boyfriend is pissed off – he had arranged to meet me at the pub and I'd forgotten. He throws me over his knee to teach me a lesson – but when he starts spanking me, it turns us both on and we end up having a simultaneous orgasm as he slaps my bottom over and over.

Belinda, 29, midwife

I'm in an old-fashioned four-poster bed with this gorgeous guy when he produces a pair of handcuffs and a whip. He puts a mask over my eyes and handcuffs me to the bed. I am breathing hard – I feel powerless to stop him from teasingly torturing me for hours. Finally, he takes off the restraints and tells me it was a test to see how much I could take and that I was amazing and he'll love me forever.

Lisa, 23, market planner

I like the idea of role-playing. Maybe playing a sweet, little innocent virgin being forced to have sex for the first time. Or maybe being an Arabian princess and have my boyfriend be my slave, having to do whatever I tell him, sexual and nonsexual. Another favourite is being raped by a gang of teenagers. Because they are young and inexperienced, I end up controlling them and teaching them how to make love. The idea of being in these situations where I have no control or total control seems sexy.

Samantha, 26, beautician

I am scared as he handcuffs my arms and legs to the bed. I don't know him that well and am putting my fate in his hands. He starts kissing me all over, his tongue reaching everywhere but my breasts and pussy. I squirm, trying to get him to go where I want, but the metal bites into my wrists and ankles. 'Stop, stay still,' he commands. 'I decide when and where to touch you.'

Scared, I stop moving. Finally, after what seems to be an eternity, he dips his head between my legs and blows lightly so that I can feel his warm breath on my clitoris. Then his tongue comes down, hard. I practically scream with relief as I come, but he keeps on kissing and licking, bringing me up again. In minutes, I come again.

This continues for what seems like hours. Finally, I cry that I can't take any more, but he tells me he decides when we're finished. Just when I think I am going to pass out from exhaustion, he climbs on top of me. If it weren't for the restraints, I would push him off. But I am caught and incredibly, I feel another orgasm building as he enters me. We both come together. He unlocks the cuffs and gently washes my skin with a scented cloth.

Selina, 27, model

You sleep deeply, but awaken when you feel my mouth on your cock. You try to reach for me, but your hands are tied to the bedposts with two of my silken scarves.

Now that you're awake, I lift my mouth from your cock, and kneel over your chest. My pussy is too far away for you to touch, although you try hard. I move back until your hard cock bumps my behind, but you aren't going to fuck me at the moment. I take a large dildo out and grease it up. I ram it into my cunt, moving it in and out, until my juices are flowing onto you.

You can feel the warmth as they flow over you. You beg me to release you, but I don't. I remove the dildo and settle my pussy over your mouth. You begin to lick my clit as I rock above you. Every once in a while I present my ass, and your tongue dives into it. I cum swiftly, the juice running down your face.

I back up and lean forward, asking you to lick and bite my hard nipples. At the same time, I reach back and begin to stroke your cock. Eventually I move back and lower myself over your cock, letting it penetrate deep into my pussy. I move up and down on your throbbing cock, until it explodes into me, our cum pooling back on the bed. I use my tongue to clean your cock, your belly, and eventually your face. I untie you and we fuck again.

Sandra, 27, marketing consultant

Bondage is something I have always wanted to try, but I am too embarrassed to tell my boyfriend Steven. In my fantasy, we are making love. He smiles at me, telling me that he has an idea. He looks in the dresser and returns with a few silk scarves. He binds me to the bed.

I struggle a little, but I want it. I half-heartedly say, 'Stop,' but Steven stops me with a kiss, murmuring that I should lie back and enjoy, because he's going to drive me wild.

He begins stroking me all over, leaving almost no place untouched. A light touch here and there, his tongue pressing against my flesh. I moan and strain against my bonds, feeling totally at his will. I can't touch him, I can't put my hands where I want them to go.

He teases me for what seems like forever before finally lowering his mouth to my vagina, his tongue pushing into me. He spreads my thighs wide, his tongue probing my clitoris. I strain against my bonds as an orgasm overtakes me.

watching
and being watched

Introduction

You are standing in front of your lover. Slowly you remove your clothes piece by piece as he watches. You feel slightly self-conscious, but also excited by the feel of his eyes on you, appreciating you, wanting you. His penis is stiff, erect, a sign of his need for you. The sight of it turns you on.

There are many variations the watching fantasy may take. Some women pretend they are a sexual performer, stripping or putting on a sex show, driving a crowd wild with their bodies and abilities. Others fantasize they are having deeply satisfying sex with someone else while their partner watches. Some women like to fantasize that they are watching someone else make love.

It's common and essentially positive for women to imagine themselves the object of lust. The attention, while put in a sexual context, is really a way of projecting oneself into the centre of attention and power – a role few women get to play in real life. The result is a feeling of well-being about oneself.

Also involved is an element of danger – especially when the fantasy involves making love in public. For many people, danger and risk are aphrodisiacs. We are most intensely excited when we're a little off-balance, uncertain, poised on the perilous edge between ecstasy and disaster. So some people like the titillation of a fantasy that involves being carried away by lust to the point where they are doing something forbidden and risk being caught.

As for fantasies about watching people make love, the idea that women aren't turned on by pornographic imagery is sexist bunk. We're all secret voyeurs – we all notice what's sexy and we like to watch sexy things. In fact, studies show that not only are women turned on by naked bodies – male and female – the market for woman-friendly X-rated movies is growing.

Whatever direction this fantasy takes, the essential thrill of these types of fantasies is of the unnoticed observer watching.

Jenny, 27, anthropologist

One of the things I love is swimming at night, but I've never been particularly brave about swimming in the nude. Last summer I was house-sitting and although the yard is fairly private, there is always a chance that someone could see me.

But one night in August when I was home alone I decided to be brave. It was hot, sticky and my swimsuit was clinging to my body as I stepped out onto the deck. I slid into the water and decided 'What the hell!' I peeled off my swimsuit and dropped it onto the deck. As I swam to the other end of the pool, I felt the water caressing my body. I had never felt anything like it ... it was kind of like being stroked with feathers all over.

This is where the fantasy takes over. I was starting to feel the effect of the water on my body. I put my hand up to one of my breasts and began to stroke my nipple, which was beginning to harden. I felt the water jet pulsing hard into my flesh ... and an idea began to form ... I faced towards the jet and slid downward until the jet just touched the lips of my pussy. The power of the jet sent shivers up and down my body. I pushed closer to the jet, and it pulsed into me. I began to move up and down, letting it pulse into me. Each time I came down I ground my hips forward on top of the jet. I wanted to come quickly because I was scared of getting caught, but at the same time, the feelings were so delicious, I wanted it to last forever.

Danielle, 27, nurse

I have never been able to fantasize during sex as I've been too involved with the man himself and my feelings. Instead, I usually play this one out when I am wanking: I own a horse farm and have advertised for summer help. The doorbell rings and there stands a tall rugged man. He asks for work, I tell him he can paint the barn.

I dress up in one of my cutest dresses that buttons all the way up the front. All day, I go out and bring him drinks and sandwiches and snacks. Each time I go out, I unbutton another button until I am just about flashing him. At the end of the day, he grabs me and practically peels the dress off my body.

We are so swept away, we don't hear the sound of approaching footsteps. It's my four farm hands – all of whom have wanted me for months. They have heard us and gathered to watch. I don't care, I am so overcome by passion. I am buck naked and putting on a show, riding the painter stranger like I would ride one of my horses. We buck and rock our way to orgasm after orgasm as everyone claps until we are both exhausted.

Clarissa, 26, designer

Although we usually have sex in bed with the lights off, in my favourite fantasy I see myself standing in front of a mirror under bright lights.

I imagine that I'm in a dressing room at a chic department store, trying on a low-cut silk dress that accents my breasts, hugs my torso, and flares out at the hips. In real life I'd never wear anything so revealing, but I look damn good in this sexy black dress. I poke my head out into the hallway and call to my lover, who has been waiting for me. I wave him into the dressing room, then I bolt the door and turn to face him. I can tell he likes what he sees. He lifts me onto a stool facing the mirrors and begins running his hands all over the dress and my body. He reaches under the dress and pulls off my lace panties. Then he ducks his head under the flared skirt and begins to kiss and lick me. My hips start to pump in a familiar rhythm that I know will lead to climax. I watch us in the mirror as we both come.

Smiling boldly, I decide to buy this dress after all.

Chrissie, 26, law student

My fiancé and I have been all over the city looking at furniture for our new apartment. We stop at my parents' house to get something to drink, and I decide to show my fiancé my old bedroom. My bed is still there, and for some reason, it turns us on to christen my old bed with my parents right below us in the kitchen. We are so hot and heavy that we don't care how much noise we are making. Suddenly, we hear my father knocking on the door. He is asking if everything is OK. We know we should stop, he is opening the door. But we can't. We are too overcome by passion. And in a back part of my mind, I realize that I am HOPING my father will see us, watch me as I climax. Which he does.

I don't know what this fantasy means. I know I don't want to make love in front of my father or have sex with him. I think it's less about sex and more about my relationship with my dad. My father has always been a very strict critical person and I think making love successfully in front of him is about my desiring some sort of approval from him.

Anonymous

My fantasy is to tell my bloke EXACTLY what I am going to do to him and to keep him in suspense as to when and where it will be. Then, when we go out in to town (somewhere nice and public!), I will discreetly wear (under my huge, long coat) some very slinky underwear. When I get 'the urge', I'll lead him to the toilet and make my move.

I'll slowly rub my body up and down him. Then, when he's nice and hard, I'll take him inside me and squeeze him to orgasm. After, we realize we never closed the door and the place is crowded with people watching us.

Sarah, 20, marketing assistant

One of my fantasies is to be working late at the office, with no-one else around and have my boyfriend come up behind me and start rubbing himself against me so he's fully aroused ... making me really wet in the process. After making me extremely horny, he would hitch my skirt up, sit me on the desk and we'd have sex on and over the desk in every position imaginable.

The next day, my boss calls me in and, placing a security videotape on the desk, says he know what happened the night before. He tells me that the only way I can save my job is to give him a blowjob. Since I secretly fancy him, this isn't as terrible as it sounds.

Before I go down on him, I ask him if he's turned off the security camera. He just smiles and I know he hasn't, that he plans to tape our daily episodes and watch them later. This just turns me on even more and I give him the best blowjob he's ever had.

Tanya, 24, receptionist

I like sex with a hint of risk, danger, the possibility of being discovered. My favourite scenario involves taking sex out of the bedroom and on the road. On a typical adventure, my boyfriend and I pack a picnic and head for the beach. We usually don't even get to the food. We look for a secluded spot, walking until no one else is visible. We spread our blanket, turn on the portable radio, and settle into each other's arms. The salt air refreshes. The sun warms. The steady wash of breaking waves sets a soothing rhythm, a relief from the city's hurrying, scurrying traffic. We cuddle, burrowing our faces into the napes of each other's necks, nibbling with little kisses.

We reach for more, fingers pressing and tongues licking all the electric places, sliding bathing suits down around our ankles. The edge is that at any moment, someone could discover us, witness our lovemaking. It's not a big risk, just enough to fuel passion and add a tingling sense of urgency.

In my fantasy, another couple stumble on us. But instead of being repulsed, they join in. Soon we are a tangle of legs, arms and mouths while the ocean laps over us.

I love to think about this fantasy – it's beautiful!

Beth, 29, hairdresser

I am walking through the park with my boyfriend when we find ourselves feeling really horny. Not being able to wait until we get home, he pulls me into the nearby bushes. We end up ripping each other's clothes off and doing it within feet of people walking by. I know they see us as my boyfriend starts sucking my nipple and fingering my snatch, and that only makes it hotter.

I want them to see, to be awed by my body and my incredible sexual prowess. I hear murmurs of approval and some clapping as I come the moment my boyfriend enters me with his stiff rod. They have never seen such a sexual creature.

After, they fall on us and ravage us – men, women, children, dogs. We are a mass of sucking and fucking and juices and smells. But I am in the centre. Everyone wants me, to touch me, to suck me, to fuck me. I come until I pass out.

I often have this fantasy while I am enjoying intercourse. Often just before coming, my eyes are closed and my fantasy gets bigger and bigger in my mind, like I'm looking at a movie screen until everything just explodes.

Lauren, 31, caterer

The stadium is filled with hundreds of men screaming and shouting. They all fall quiet as she steps forward into the spotlight. She's dressed in a floor length gown, shoulders bare, auburn hair swept atop her head. Her earrings dangle as her green eyes sweep the crowd, daring anyone to say anything. Madonna's *Like A Virgin* starts playing. She begins to dance, arms over head. Then her hands drop to her neck, fingers stroking inside the top of her dress. She slips her hand lower, stroking her nipple through the silky material of the dress. It hardens instantly and some of the men sigh. She can feel their eyes burning into her as she slides her hand down her body, pressing hard against her mound, through the dress. She moans softly, and the audience, anticipating what is going to come next, moan with her. Her hands reaches for the dress's side zipper and suddenly, the dress falls to the floor and she is standing there naked. She sways to the music as she hears the sound of them all coming, coming, in tribute to her.

'She' is really me, but I envision the whole thing in the third person. In another fantasy I have, I imagine I am on a stage, masturbating in front of a roomful of guys. They are cheering me on. My hand moves faster and faster. Everyone comes when I do.

Rachel, 26, Nurse

My fantasies have kept me going through a very bad time and kept me sane. I was sexually abused by my first husband. After years of awful horrific sex and being told I was terrible in bed, I believed it. My next partner was a 'safe house' but I was never able to have an orgasm with him. Finally, after years of bad sex, I had a relationship with a man who taught me I wasn't a freak and gave me sexual liberation.

But through all the bad years, one fantasy kept me going and helped me to believe I wasn't frigid. I would lie in the bath, close my eyes and imagine that I was in a big open room, totally empty expect for a large one-way mirror. On the outside would be a gathering of gorgeous men. I somehow knew they were there and would feel very self-conscious but titillated about lying there, naked and exposed except for a few bubbles.

Slowly, I would start to stroke myself, starting from my head and gradually working my way down. The thought of being watched as I bring myself to orgasm is totally erotic. Because there was no way the men could get in and touch me gave me a feeling of incredible power.

Even though I have now 'awakened', and I have more fantasies, this one is special to me.

Nadine, 22, PA

My fantasy has always been to make sensual hot love at the back of a limousine. It's summer and we're stuck in traffic with the sun-roof open but the windows are tinted and closed. My lover slowly strips me, making love to each body part as it becomes exposed.

First, he kisses my lips. Then he licks his way down to my shoulders and arms and sucks each finger. He spends a long time on my breasts, biting and nibbling at them. Then he trails his tongue down my stomach, sending shivers throughout my body. Finally, he dips into my honey pot, sucking and eating while I buck with joy. Just when I think I can't take any more, he continues down my legs to my toes and back up to my backside where he swirls his tongue. I cry as I come.

Throughout all this, we are creating a traffic jam as drivers are curious to know what is happening in the limo that is bucking and shaking. I am turned on knowing that we're doing it and no one can see us but we can see them.

Just writing this letter is making me feel horny.

Maria, 27, teacher

I like being watched. The thrill of someone looking on makes me wet. One night when my husband and I went out to dinner I pulled his cock out and started stroking it. There were people all around. It seemed to make us both hornier. We saved coming for later on when we got home. Another time he went down on me while we were at a park. This time I got to come. WOW, what an orgasm!!! I would like to try watching. Someday.

Anna, 28, shop manager

I love to have someone turn the lights off and then take a flashlight and shine it directly on my pussy and watch while they finger me. I could let someone do this for hours. Thinking about this makes me orgasm over and over.

I also fantasize about standing in the window and masturbating while the man next door watches. It feels so good to think that when I touch myself, he is watching me.

Another fantasy I have is that my husband watches while I make love to another woman. I don't know who she is, but she looks a lot like me. We could be sisters. I nuzzle her breasts and finger her clitoris, making her moan with pleasure. Meanwhile, my husband is watching us and rubbing his penis. I know he wants to join us, but he can't. I don't know why, but he isn't allowed to move. The blissful moment comes when I go down on the woman and we all start coming together.

Anonymous

I would love to watch my husband fuck someone hot in the ass. I don't know why. I have no desire to be fucked in the ass by him. But the image of his penis, rock hard, sinking in and out of someone with a beautiful creamy white, fleshy bum is indescribably sexy to me.

Becky, 32, lab technician

I love the idea of watching my boyfriend jack off. To see him cum would be very exciting for me. Then he would watch me take care of myself – sometimes with just my fingers and other times with my vibrator.

I think this is a fantasy I might share with him someday. I am not sure if he would be intimidated by the idea of me giving myself an orgasm or take my fantasy to mean that I think I can take care of myself better than he can. I hope not because that's not true at all. He's a great lover. It's just that I get so into having sex that sometimes I feel like I am missing out on the EXPERIENCE of it all and watching would give me the chance to just sit back and enjoy the show of sex.

Erin, 24, personal assistant

Having had a long day I decide to check out a new women's club that I'd heard about from a friend. She said it was exactly as you would picture a Roman bath. Columns surrounded a central pool, and doors opened to rooms off to the side for other diversions ... sauna, massage, and a steam room.

I have never been in a steam room like this. It is like something you would see in a movie, or perhaps a fantasy ...

A stack of towels sits just outside the door. Stone benches are scattered around the good sized room, and a few naked or semi-naked women are relaxing inside. I remove my swimsuit and put a towel on one of the benches and lay down on my back. I look around to see what is going on.

Nothing much.

The hot steam in the room relax me quickly, the tension flowing from me. I see two women near me, one blonde, the other brunette. They don't see me because of the steam. The blonde gets up and puts the 'Closed for Cleaning' sign on the door. Suddenly, in a room full of heat and moisture, my throat is dry.

She smiles and goes back to her friend. The brunette is now on her back, her legs hanging over the sides of the bench. The blonde straddles the bench, between her legs. Her hands reach out and caress her lover's body, with a touch that comes from knowing the intimate details of someone. You can see the brunette's face contort with passion as fingers stroke her favourite places. The blonde leans over and presses her lips down on top of the brunette's. As the kiss is broken I can see her tongue sliding from the other woman's mouth.

Her fingers brush against her lover's pussy, just barely touching the shaved mound. The brunette's back arches upwards, trying to make contact. Using one hand, the blonde spreads her wider, one finger sliding deep into her wetness. Small moans come from the brunette's lips.

She slides two fingers slowly into the brunette, her pace increasing slightly. The brunette is lifting her pelvis to meet each stroke, and soon a third finger joins the other two. The blonde's mouth teases her clit, causing her to cry out with her climax. I can see as she lifts her mouth away that four fingers are now pumping furiously in and out of the brunette's cunt.

Another orgasm begins. As she bucks on the bench I can see the blonde's entire hand slide into the brunette's cunt. It seems now that the brunette is coming non-stop, her screams of ecstasy filling the room, echoing off the walls. The blonde finally slows her pace and slides her hand and fingers out of the brunette, letting her collapse against the bench, murmuring words of love in her ear.

I come just watching them.

Catherine, 31, scientist

I often turn to fantasy with my husband to jump-start my sexual energy. In one of my favourite fantasies, I imagine that as I hug a close girlfriend of mine, a man watches us from a comfortable chair in the corner of their living room. He's a stranger, a straight man getting more and more excited by watching us.

I imagine that we tease him, saying things like, 'Have you ever had two girls at the same time?' But we also control him. He can't do a thing, he can't even leave his chair, unless we give him permission.

His desire gets more and more intense until he's ready to explode. At that point, I usually forget all about the fantasy man and concentrate instead on mutual stimulation in real-life with my partner.

SEX FANTASIES BY WOMEN FOR WOMEN

My fantasy has fulfilled its function: to awaken and enhance my interest in sex.

Annette, 27, market researcher

Sometimes when my husband and I make love, I get off by thinking that a man is looking through the window and watching. It makes sex more exciting if I imagine my lover and I are on a stage making love. Many people watch us and get aroused.

During sex, I like to think that several men are standing and watching my partner and me. These men get very turned on and take their dicks out – but never participate with us.

Jenny, 30, assistant producer

I fantasize about making a porn film with my boyfriend. The idea of all these people watching us to turn on is a total turn on for me. It drives me to do things I normally never would, like suck my boyfriend and swallow. Everyone is very disappointed that they don't see my boyfriend come. But then I stick my bum out to my boyfriend, inviting him to stick his penis in – something my boyfriend has been urging me to do but I can't see myself ever doing in real life. But now, it is something I want, I need. The people watching cheer and urge me on. I circle my bum around my boyfriend's stiff stick. Meanwhile, he has reached around and is playing with my breasts and stroking my clit. Everyone is masturbating now, even the camera people. The room smells of sex. We all come together.

Anna, 32, events organizer

My husband and I are both sitting on the bed, my legs over his, both of us with legs spread wide. While I lean back on one hand and play with my breasts and pussy, he watches me and while he watches me, he strokes his cock. We both get to watch each other play with ourselves, trying hard to hold off from touching the other until we both come.

This fantasy always makes me come in about a second.

Janet, 28, flight attendant

I love the idea of opening my legs and stroking myself for anyone who wants to watch. Soon a crowd gathers. I work myself very slowly, sliding my hands up and down and around my clitoris. I let the pressure build. The people watching – they are mainly faceless and sexless, just a large group I sense is there – are urging me to let myself go. They want me to have my orgasm, need me to have it. Finally I can't hold back any longer. My climax shoots out with such force it looks like a geyser. Everyone cheers.

Paula, 32, DJ

We just moved into a new condo recently and the unit across our common driveway has blinds but they are never shut. A young woman, probably in her late 20s, owns the place. Our bedrooms are directly across from each other. She gets in from work very late but I fight to stay awake so I can see her undress and walk naked into her master bathroom which is also very visible. She usually puts the blinds down at this point, but in my fantasy, when she comes back in, I can see her large breasts and hairy pussy. She is fleshy and big, like me. I am naked with the blinds up and all the lights on. I hope she sees me, but she doesn't. She starts to caress herself. I can see her fingers dipping in and out of her pussy and mine match her. Faster and faster,

SEX FANTASIES BY WOMEN FOR WOMEN

harder and harder. We come together. She lies there, recovering, still completely unaware of me.

Jacqueline, 31, aromatherapist

I use this fantasy during sex with my husband and when I'm masturbating. It always gives me an orgasm. During the fantasy, I'm still the same person except I have this really beautiful body. My breasts are perfect and my tight body has no fat.

I imagine I'm a stripper in a really high-class place. I'm the top-billed dancer and everyone in the audience can't wait until I begin dancing. My costume is a beautiful golden bikini with sparkles, sequins and white diamonds sewn on. I'm wearing a white-feathered headband and four-inch gold high heels with white feather plumes on the top. I use a beautiful, long, white feather boa to tease the audience while I'm stripping to the beat of the music. All eyes are on me and the men's jaws are open because they can't believe how beautiful I am. The men all want me and they're begging me to take it off!

I slowly unfasten my bikini top and hide my breasts behind the feather boa. The top drops to the floor so everyone realises my breasts are exposed, I move the feathers around and around, still covering myself. Slowly, slowly I let the boa drop to the floor and there I am. I'm topless in front of the cheering audience.

The men in the front row stand to get a better look at me. One man can't help himself, he's so overcome with desire for me, he comes over as if he's hypnotized by me and he reaches a hand in the air, as if to touch me. I like his look – which is a lot like my husband's – so I dance over to him. He reaches up and gently runs his hand over my body.

All of a sudden it's just this man and me. He's gentle but insistent in his desire for me and I decide to let him have me. He lays me down on the stage and kisses my breasts. I'm so turned on, I'm ready to explode and he finally makes beautiful love to me right there on the stage. I try to get up because I remember the audience is watching us, but he is such a fantastic lover – nuzzling my neck, caressing my flat belly, tickling my thighs – that I lose the will to move. The audience is clapping as we make incredible passionate love.

I usually use this thought to masturbate by – and sometimes to climax during intercourse. Usually, my mind races ahead to the finish and skips all the details so I climax before I get much beyond the stripping scene.

Rachel, 25, pharmacist

I am making a video with my boyfriend. I eat him, he eats me, he penetrates me and we go to town. The turn-on is that every moment is being filmed for a worldwide audience and I know they will be beating themselves off while watching me get off.

The lights are bright and hot. Many people are standing around photographing and directing. Everyone is very excited by my body, my movements.

I am the most sensuous woman in the world, I love being the centre of sexual attention and know that every man who sees this film will want me and every woman will want to be me because I clearly know how to please a man and myself. My boyfriend makes me come and come again and the audience goes wild.

Beth, 27, therapist

I imagine I'm watching a man and woman make love. He's a man I used to know, but have never slept with. The woman is someone in my neighbourhood I think – she is vaguely familiar. It's unimportant because she then becomes me, although I am somehow still watching us from the outside.

He's very, very gentle. He has an erection before he's undressed. I finished undressing him and then he undresses me. Our bodies come together and I rub against his penis. He leads me toward the bed, pushes me down gently and begins to play with me. After a while, I tell him I'm ready for him to enter me. He rolls over, his penis quivering straight up.

I watch myself mount him, slide his organ into me, and rock back and forth until we both climax.

I think about this fantasy several times a month, usually during masturbation though sometimes during sex if it seems I am not going to come fast enough. I've had it for several years. It started when I happened to see a friend of mine make love with some guy when we were sharing a hotel room on holiday. But the main element for me is the man's utter gentleness. He is so considerate of me.

Phillipa, 32, managing director

I am on a beach somewhere in the Caribbean. It is a nude beach. So I spread my towel out and remove my bathing suit.

I lay in the sun for a while feeling the heat on my body. Worried about burning, I reach for the suntan lotion. I spread the warm cream into my hand and spread it over my legs and arms. Realizing now that I have other areas to cover, I begin to spread the lotion over my stomach and upwards to my breasts.

My nipples harden as I stroke the lotion over my breasts. I pinch one nipple lightly, feeling a rush of pleasure run up my spine. My hands continue to caress my body, no longer caring if I have any lotion on them. My fingers slide between my legs, one finger sliding deep into my pussy. I pull it out and push two fingers deep inside.

I see two men nearby watching me, and I admit I am thrilled by the fact that they are watching. My thumb rubs my clit slowly, as I gently push a third finger into my pussy. I arch upward as my orgasm hits, the warm liquid flowing from my cunt and running between the cheeks of my ass.

I lay back down on the towel, feeling the slow come-down from my orgasm. I stay there for a while, just stroking my body lightly now and then. The men have disappeared and I lie there, working on my tan.

Tiffany, 25, hairstylist

One brisk fall day, several of my friends decide to enjoy the day at some nearby wineries. After a few bottles of great wine, my boyfriend and I decide to take a walk. We stop at a spot behind an old barn that has been turned into a shop that's closed for the season. In unspoken consensus, we fall to the ground and have the greatest sex ever. My fantasy now is that the shop is open and everyone can see us. When we are finished, they applaud.

Amanda, 27, bike-shop manager

In the summer, my favourite activity is going fishing with my now ex-boyfriend. We spend up to five hours a day out on the water in a boat, talking, fishing, swimming. In this fantasy, he asks me to pass him a beer. When I get closer to him, he starts to massage my rear end. Before I know it, he has his shorts off, I have my bikini bottom off, and we are making love in the middle of the lake. It's especially exciting because I wonder if anyone can see us from their lake home or a passing boat.

Terri, 28, computer programmer

My husband is a physician and usually very conservative when it comes to public displays of affection. My fantasy is that on a trip to Mexico (where we spent our honeymoon), he is willing to be a bit more daring. We are on a sightseeing tour bus and he begins touching me. Then he slips his hand under my skirt and pleasures me until I reach orgasm. I let out a yelp and fake a yawn when the older couple sitting in front of us turn around. I don't know if the excitement is the idea that my husband is being outrageous or that we are doing this on a bus full of people!

Jillian, 26, finance manager

I'm waiting for my boyfriend, who is late. I am dressed in a black lace teddy, and had planned a surprise. I was going to open the door in it and spiked heels. I can feel the lace of the bra rubbing against my nipples, making them hard.

I reach in and touch my breast, stroking it. I suck on a finger and run it around the nipple until it is hard. I reach down and free my other breast, doing the same to it. I run my hands down my legs, stroking them, bring my fingers to my mound. I undo the snaps of the teddy, slipping my fingers in.

I'm very wet. I decide there is no reason to wait. I get up slowly and go into the bedroom closet for my box of toys (I don't own a box of toys, but always thought it would be a sexy thing to have). I select two items, one a huge lifelike cock with two ends, and the other a small vibrator just a little thicker than my finger. I turn the base on the vibrator just to make sure the batteries are still fresh, which they are. I turn it off for the moment. I lift the large cock and bring it to my mouth. I run my tongue over the head, wetting it with my saliva.

When it is finally glistening, I lower it and slowly begin to push the head into my wet waiting hole. I push it in as far as it will go, only halfway, and stop for a minute to enjoy how full I feel. I begin to move it slowly in and out, bringing the tip almost completely out before plunging it back in. I feel my orgasm building and decide to help it over the top. I pick up the vibrator and touch it lightly to my clit. The reaction is almost immediate. I climax fast and hard, a cry escaping my lips as I fall backwards against the couch.

I lie there for a minute stroking my breasts, thinking how glad I am that my boyfriend is late. Then I feel someone watching me. It is my boyfriend, standing in the door. He has witnessed my entire orgasm. He strips and we make passionate love.

Katherine, 25, data programmer

I am very much into the whole voyeur side of sex. I'd like to do a strip tease and lap dance for my boyfriend ... in front of a lot of people! The idea of sex out on a beach where there are a lot of people around is a turn-on for me.

Dana, 28, retail manager

We are making love. I met him at a club and we were drawn to each other immediately. His tongue licks at my thighs, causing me to spasm. He comes up and kisses me. I can taste myself in our kiss. My hands roam his body, exploring. My mouth tastes him ... his lips, his neck, his shoulder, his nipple, his stomach, his thigh, his cock. I engulf him with one thrust, pulling him into my warm wet mouth, feeling him throb within me. I pull my head away and move upward. I want to feel his cock deep within me. I spread my legs, position him, and lower myself onto him. I feel his hard cock sliding deep into me, filling me. I begin to move, rocking against him. As I lean over him, my breasts brushing his chest, I see his eyes widen at something over his shoulder. I turn to look and see a tall brunette in a business outfit watching us. She looks pissed off.

I realise it is his wife and know I should leave, but suddenly, I can feel him coming and I begin coming too. She watches as we collapse, completely spent.

Sindi, 27, independent film director

I love to fantasize when I'm masturbating. My favourite has a bunch of people in a room. No one has any clothes on. There are two Nordic-looking women kissing. A man joins them and begins caressing their bodies. He is dark and the contrast between their bodies is striking. There's a deep, sexy beat playing in the background and the three grind sensuously against each other in time to the music. One of the women drops to her knees and begins sucking the man's rock-hard penis. He groans and thrusts himself deep into her mouth. The other woman crawls behind her friend and begins licking her pussy while fingering herself. The music gets louder and faster as they get build towards their climax. Finally, just as I explode, they all come in one fantastic orgasm.

Ina, 26, stock controller

I am watching two gay guys have sex while I masturbate. Their faces are never clear, but their bodies are long and thin. They don't see me. I watch as the taller one's penis slides in and out of the other's bum hole. The one who is getting fucked is stroking himself. Meanwhile, I'm rubbing myself hard. We orgasm at the same time.

Tara, 29, graphic artist

I go to an art gallery on my own and while I'm wandering around, I spot this fantastic looking man staring at a nude statue. He's very arty with long hair and a black shirt unbuttoned so I can see hair sprouting from his chest. I imagine he has to have me right there and then. I get turned on by the idea of people watching us as we make love.

Sometimes when I'm having sex, I imagine my lover and I are in front of the window and people walking by are looking in.

Suzanne, 27, surveyor

I'm in bed one night, half asleep, and I hear you enter the apartment. It's surprising as I'm not expecting you. I'm about to get up and see why you're here, when I hear you talking to someone ... you're obviously not alone. I lie quietly on the bed with my eyes closed as the bedroom door opens and you come in. I hear you telling the person you're with to be quiet, as I'm asleep.

You approach the bed, removing the covers gently. You expose my naked body to your friend, who comments about my sleeping nude. I know now that you have brought another man home with you. I feel a hand touch me gently and stroke down my arm. I pretend to shift in my sleep, I am on my side now, legs slightly apart. The hand strokes my breast lightly, focusing on the nipple, as another hand lightly touches my vaginal lips.

I moan slightly, and the hands move away immediately. You assure him that it won't matter if I'm awake, but he's not sure if he should believe you. Still pretending to be asleep, I begin to touch myself. One hand slowly explores my breasts, pinching and rubbing my nipples until they are hard. The other hand slides between my legs, parting my lips, probing my vaginal lips. I start to moan again, moving my hand faster in and out of my wet vagina. The two of you have stopped talking and I know you are watching. The hand on my breasts slides over my side and towards my ass, one finger probing my anus. The other hand in my pussy is plunging in and out, my thumb rubbing my clit. I climax hard, juices flowing over my hand.

Janet, 25, PR assistant

I am at a bar. A couple are on a stage. They begin with a kiss, soft at first, then deepening into a searing embrace. He undoes her top, tossing it aside. Then his mouth lowers to her breast, capturing her nipple.

As his hands slide slowly under the edge of her skirt, she presses hard against him, tearing at his clothes. They both manage to pull the material from one another, leaving them naked before us. He turns her over and lowers her to the platform, spreading her wide. His head dips between her legs, and she begins to moan.

I glance around at the audience, mainly to see their reactions. Most have slid hands beneath their clothing, touching themselves. As the woman on the dais continues to moan, even louder now, I find my hand sliding between the folds of my skirt, stroking. I watch now as the man stands behind her, slowly pushing his cock deep inside her.

I watch as a member of the audience approaches them, dropping her clothing on the floor, and kneeling between their legs. Her tongue darts out to lick his balls, and her clit, in turn. Another member of the audience approaches, a man this time. He's naked. He stands in front of the first woman, his hard cock within reach of her mouth.

The first man climaxes, his semen pouring from his cock into the mouth of the woman below, who pulls his still pulsing cock into her mouth. The first woman pulls the other man's cock deeply into her mouth, and he begins to pump in and out of her.

The woman below her begins to suck hard on her clit, her efforts soon rewarded by gushing juices that covers her face. She leans back and watches the other woman sucking the cock, pressing her fingers deep into her own pussy. The second man comes in a burst, filling the woman's mouth with his hot, sticky juices.

They move aside, watching the lone woman fingering herself. She has three fingers pumping in and out of herself, her thumb rubbing her clit. She brings a single finger to her mouth, wetting it. She moves slightly, pushes her finger deep in her anus, her orgasm taking her then. She lays still for a minute, and the audience claps heartily and I climax at the same time, collapsing against the couch, breathing quickly.

a walk
on the wild side

Introduction

Imagine one mouth caressing your lips, another sucking your nipple, a third nuzzling your genitals, while six hands touch your body all at once.

There are some things you may have thought about trying out sexually that you wouldn't dream of sharing with your lover. Fear of rejection stops you from mentioning anything like anal sex, sex with another man, a fling with his best friend or even him and your best friend.

These fantasies are about sexual curiosity, pure and simple. They allow you to mentally let your hair down, be yourself, show off, do whatever you want with your body and be desired no matter what. Women often mentally conjure up multiple partners as a way to multiply the sources of sexual stimulation they receive. How else are you ever going to experience oral sex and vaginal penetration at the same time?

Other favourite plots in the wild theme include being a prostitute or a stripper, having sex in some spot where there's a risk of being caught, being in a sex video. Believe it or not, there is nothing weird about these fantasies – they're usually triggered by something that happened to you in childhood, or puberty when you're first discovering what turns you on.

What these fantasies have in common is that they allow you to get into all sorts of exploration, free from any of the hassles of commitment. It's a totally impersonal yet completely fulfilling encounter, and the fact that these are fantasies few women would want to carry out in real-life only adds to the excitement. Plus the sex for sale angle means you're in control, which is why this is often the preferred fantasy of women who tend to have poor sexperiences with men in real life or who find it hard to express themselves in their day-to-day life. Here, you're the one calling the shots – and he has to play by your rules. You get to be the ultimate sex queen, surrounded by men who are driven wild by your erotic antics but can only look and never touch – unless you say so.

Diane, 31, web-page designer

My husband and I celebrated our fifth anniversary at a cosy bed-and-breakfast. In my fantasy, I plan to try something sexually new that weekend. As I dress for the trip, I also pack our video camera. After dinner, back in our room, I take out the camera, turn it on, and walk into the living room of our suite, where my husband is waiting, nude. The camera makes him a little shy at first, but I get him in the mood when I lift my skirt. He puts the camera on the table, and it records every hot moment of our lovemaking. We spend the rest of the weekend replaying the video and having wild, passionate sex, again and again.

I have this fantasy when I am extremely turned on and then it helps bring me to a really good orgasm.

Molly, 26, advertising executive

I am in bed naked with two men. I don't know who they are. Both are very good-looking.

I point to one and tell him to taste my juices. He slides his fingers between my legs and sucks them, one at a time. His penis swells. It's huge. I can hardly wait.

I suck both of their cocks a little, making them rock-hard.

I straddle one of the men, mounting him quickly. I slide him deep into my vagina, gasping as he fills me with his hot, throbbing cock. I push myself down onto his cock, letting it fill me completely. I begin to move up and down on it, gripping hard with my vaginal muscles, enjoying the sensations of his cock. I lean over him and press my body against his, covering his chest with my mouth, licking, sucking, biting.

I feel the other man moving in close behind me, his hands stroking my bum. 'Go on, fuck me in there. Do it,' I implore. I reach back and spread the cheeks wide, giving him easy access to my bum-hole. He wets his fingers and spreads his saliva over the entrance to my bum, pressing one finger in gently. With more lubrication he manages to get two fingers in. 'Go on, put it in, now,' I order. He slowly pushes it in. 'Harder, harder,' I beg, as he starts moving in and out.

Both men keep their pace slow, knowing what it is doing to me. I start moaning. Their pace increases. They plunge in and out of me at a furious pace. As my orgasm builds, the one fucking me in the bum suddenly pulls out and splashes his cum all over my ass and the other man's body. I rub it in, licking my hands occasionally. The other man comes and I quickly follow.

The men disappear and I am left there, fully satiated.

Claire, 21, therapist

I masturbate frequently, ever since I first had sex. I find it does nothing for me unless I fantasize. This is one I often have: I've been working late again. I leave the office and think of what to do. My boyfriend is out of town and I've been horny all day. I pass a bar on the way home and decide to stop in for a drink. There are two men sitting down at the end of the bar, looking me over. I order a scotch, straight up. I decide to have some fun, so I run my lips over the rim of the glass before taking a drink. The two guys can't stop staring, and I'm beginning to get into it. They talk between themselves. I know they're arguing over who is going to try and pick me up ... if only they knew.

I slide down from the stool and approach them. I lean in close and say softly, 'You don't have to fight. You can both fuck me.' The blonde just stares, but his dark-haired friend says, 'My place is nearby – let's go.' Once in his flat, we head for the bedroom. I have one of them unzip my dress and I slip it off. I walk over to the blonde and slowly help him off with his clothes. I put his penis in my mouth and feel it grow hard in my mouth. I leave him for a minute and undress his friend. He's already starting to harden.

I stand them side-by-side and start to go down on them. My head goes back and forth between them until they are both hard. I lie on the bed and ask one of them to lick my pussy. The brunette quickly kneels between my legs, his tongue sliding and swirling over me, making me wet. His friend licks and bites my breasts and nipples.

Finally, I feel I'm ready. I tell the blonde to lie on the bed and I lower my wet pussy over him. I take some spit and rub it over my bum-hole. The brunette sticks one finger in, then two. Once I'm stretched, he positions his cock at the head of my anus and pushes forward. I can't believe the ecstasy as I am filled with two hard penises. I begin to move up and down on the penis below me as the other penis drives in and out of my bum. I lose track of how many times I come. The man in my bum pulls out of me and climaxes over my back, rubbing his juices into me. I can feel the penis below me swelling to orgasm as I come again.

Lisa, 29, anthropologist

I usually start fantasizing when my lover penetrates me. There are two men – Tim and James, the boyfriends of two of my friends – with me. The funny thing is I wouldn't want to sleep with them in real life, but in my fantasies, they seem really sexy. I take turns sucking them deep into my mouth, licking their cocks, probing their balls. Tim lies down on the bed and I position myself over him, sliding down on his cock. He grabs me firmly and helps me move up and down on his cock. James positions himself behind me, his cock pressing against my bum. He pushes in slowly, filling me completely. The two of them begin to fuck me almost in a rhythm. I mentally pace it so we – meaning me in real life! – come just as my lover has his orgasm.

Nora, 26, credit controller

I find masturbating while in my car a total turn-on ... and yes, even better with the sun shining on my spread legs. I often need to drive into the City for a meeting, it's a 20-minute drive, and when I'm in the mood, I slip out my hand between my legs, and slowly jerk off ... sometimes I cum, sometimes I hold off until I park ...

I'm not too sure if anyone has spotted me, but it's a total turn-on to fantasize that I could be seen.

Claire, 28, waitress

I used to commute a half an hour to work and most of the drive was motorway driving. I worked the late shift, and to keep myself awake on my way back home, I would masturbate almost the whole way back home. I would fantasize that a cop pulled me over and in order to avoid a ticket, I had to give him a blowjob. A similar fantasy was that I broke down and had to fuck the repairman or a passing motorist who offered to help me.

I would have to be careful to hold back until there were no other cars around when I came. Sometimes when I came, and my back arched and my head went back onto my shoulders, I would swerve a little into the other lane.

I never cared if truckers or whoever saw, although I did usually just have my hands down in my pants, so I guess it would have been tougher to see since I still had all my clothes on.

Looking back, it would have been nice to have had a guy to carpool with. I would have loved keeping a guy awake by sucking his cock while he drove, and letting him finger my pussy and suck my tits while I drove.

Kim, 31, credit controller

Sometimes, when I start to masturbate, I run my hands up and down my body, feeling the curves and proud that I have taken care of my body. I caress my soft skin and play with my breasts – almost as if I'm tantalizing someone to have sex with me. In this way, I start to become sexually excited about my own body. This can even be better if I lie in front of a mirror and spread my legs. Then I start thinking about this: I'm walking the street at night. A car pulls up and we make a deal. The man drives on. He puts his hand between my legs and gives me an orgasm. I sometimes have this fantasy while driving and have to pull off while I come.

Jane, 31, junior doctor

I am home alone watching some old porn movie I have on video and I'm getting turned on as I strip down to nothing. I lay on the floor naked, with a pillow beneath my head and a blanket over me. I'm following what the woman does, but pretending the man there is Mike, my boyfriend. Smiling behind her as he butt-fucks her. At the same time, my pussy grows nice and warm and wet and I touch myself, humping the pillow beneath me, until I orgasm.

Louisa, 31, travel agent

I never have an orgasm unless I am masturbating. In my fantasy, I find this service that promises to give you one over the phone. Hesitantly, I call the number.

'Hello?' I whisper into the phone.

'Hello,' says a deep male voice. 'I want you to get a few things before we start if you will. A bowl of ice cubes, a cold drink for you and a hand mirror. No questions, just do as I ask please. When you get back to your room I want you to set those items next to your bed and get completely undressed.'

I do as he says and tell him.

'Good. Try and relax. Get the mirror and use it to slowly view your whole body. Start at your face and describe your skin, then move down to your neck, chest and breasts. Tell me what you see.'

I feel funny, but I do as he orders. 'My breasts are firm and rounded. The skin seems whiter on my breasts, almost translucent. My areola is dark pink and my nipples are small. I've seen some pictures of ladies who have nipples that stick way out but mine don't do that.'

'That's good ... keep going ... over your stomach now and down to your genital area and legs.'

'My stomach is fairly flat. My pubic hair starts just under my stomach. It's not very thick and is brown and curly. My thighs are a little flabby I guess, but my calves are muscular and shapely. My feet are just feet.'

'You're doing very well,' says the voice. 'Now bend your knees, and put your feet flat on the bed just under the cheeks of your butt. Spread your knees apart and rest the phone on your shoulder. Then take one hand and gently open the lips to your vagina. Spread them slightly, just enough to describe what you see inside. I'm sure it looks like a beautiful flower. Can you see your clitoris? Is it poking out of the hood?'

I feel funny looking at myself – something I have never done before – but something about the voice compels me not to disobey. My lips are spread slightly and deep pink folds protrude from either side. It resembles a flower, like an orchid. Near the top of the opening is my clitoris. I tell him all this.

'Good. Now spread yourself open using only one hand. Take your index finger from your other hand and get it very wet in your mouth. When it is very wet take your finger and circle your clitoris. Don't touch it directly, just make nice soft circles around the hood. Are you doing that now?'

'Yes,' I breathe.

'Think about how you're feeling. Concentrate on the sensations you're creating. Keep making the circles, and if you start to get dry, lick your finger again. That's it, I can hear your breathing change a little. That must be starting to feel real good now. I want you to stop now and gently massage the folds of your vagina while you tell me what you are feeling.'

I don't want to stop, but I do, knowing the conversation would end if he thinks I am not following his instructions. 'It started way down inside me ... kind of a tingling. It spread through my insides and then across my skin. It is really incredible and I feel wet.'

'It's time to concentrate on your breasts for a while. Keep the phone in the crook of your neck and take both of your index fingers and just barely touch the tip of your nipple. Now with the slightest pressure, and without lifting them ... rotate them the tiniest bit. Use the tip of your fingernail to just barely tease the nipple tip. Are your nipples getting hard?'

'Ooh, that feels so good.'

'Keep doing what I tell you. Don't talk to me now. Take an ice cube and lightly rub it over your nipples. Make circles with the ice all over your breasts. That's it. Nice and slow. I know that feels good. Get another cube as that one melts. Till the ice is all gone. Now take your hand and flatten it. Spread it out so the palm is very stiff. Now just barely scrape your nipples with your palm. That's it, keep going. Now push your palm flat against your breast and knead your whole breast in your hands. Use your thumb and forefinger to roll and then lightly pinch your nipples. Ahh! I can hear you moaning now – don't stop.

'I'm starting to get aroused too. My cock is very hard now. I've unzipped my pants and have my cock in my hand now. I'm stroking it slowly and every now and them I lick my thumb and rub it across the glans. That feels so good. I imagine it's you.

'Keep rolling your nipples. Can you feel the sensations all the way to your clitoris? I imagine it's your hand stroking me and you licking me.

'Oh God, baby, that feels so good. Keep one hand on your breasts and move the other down to your pussy. I want you to start making those circles again. Use your own juices this time to wet your fingers. I can tell from the way you are breathing you're very wet. Take your other fingers and put them just inside the lips. Move them slightly in and out and side to side. Ohh, that's it, baby. I can tell that feels good, doesn't it?'

I can hardly breathe. 'Oh my God,' I cry, 'something is happening ...'

'Don't stop ... keep going ... that's it ... don't stop. You're almost there. Yes ... oh God, I'm going to come with you, baby ... do it NOW – DO IT!'

'Ohhh! YES!!!!!!'

'I can hear you breathing ... are you OK honey? Say something.'

I laugh and say, 'You can call me twice a day!'

Natalie, 30, actress

I fantasize dozens of times a day and each fantasy is very different. If there are recurring themes, they are based on group sex and wild sex; things I wouldn't necessarily do. In the last one I had, I am invited to a party in the street where I live. When I arrive, I find a load of couples getting it on with each other. I think about leaving but then decide to join in. I end up being the most popular person in the room with people lining up to get off with me.

Dana, 31, management consultant

I agree to go with my boyfriend to his boss's party. As we walk through the door, I see groups of two, three, even four people kissing and fondling each other and I realize this isn't an ordinary drinks party. I look at my boyfriend as if to say, 'Did you know about this' and he just grins and starts kissing me. I feel someone behind me caressing my bum. I don't know if it's a man or a woman. Someone else reaches and lifts my dress over my head and slides my pants down. I am now completely naked. Hands and mouths touch and lick at my body. A penis grazes my cheek and I start sucking on it. I run my tongue over the head, pulling him in deeper. Someone is biting my clitoris and the same person – or is it someone else – is fingering my bum. Juices trickle from me and my hips arch involuntarily as I come. I feel someone – is it a man? It MUST be a man – pushing me back and positioning himself between my legs. He pushes in hard, causing a gasp from me. I take him deep inside of me and we both explode. I open my eyes and find myself looking into my boyfriend's eyes.

Suzanna, 28, stock broker

I am swimming in a lake by myself. I am nude. I feel exhilarated, sexy, strong and free.

Swimming back to the shore, I lie down on a boulder, letting the sun and mountain air dry me. The air moves over my skin. I part my legs to allow the breeze access to the most intimate parts of my body. It feels like silk, moving over my feet, dipping down between my legs, whispering to my pussy, my ass, following the contours of the lips, poking between the cheeks, then up my tummy, blowing on my breasts, swirling around the erect nipples, tumbling down to the hollows of my neck and shoulders, then over my face and hair.

I lay very still, my breathing changing as I feel the quickening between my legs and in the pit of my stomach. I let the sensation grow slowly, not moving, allowing the mountain air to whisper to my body. Without even touching myself, I feel myself getting moist, and a low, contented moan escapes from my lips. I don't know how long I can keep my hands from my body, but I want to prolong this delicious ravishment as long as I can. I spread my legs even further, opening myself to the wind.

The breeze becomes fingers, hundreds of little fingers, and tongues, hundreds of minuscule, warm tongues, moving over my body, lifting the fine hairs on my tummy and breasts and arms, rustling through the triangle of soft fur between my legs, pushing here, licking there, inserting themselves into my vagina, my anus, tasting the sensitive skin of my inner thighs, insistently probing the lips of my pussy, blindly seeking the kernel of my clit. I open my legs even more, bending and lifting my knees to allow the wind access to the moisture, to the growing, hardening bud at the top of my pussy. The tongues of air seem to spread open the outer lips, then the softer inner lips, then caress my clit with warm vibrations. The fingers enter me, moving in and out of my every opening. Tongues and fingers reaching my very core, tickling my navel, up to my breasts, my fully erect nipples strain for more, more.

Time is meaningless. Minutes pass, hours, days. My breathing becomes tiny whimpers. I moan with the immense pressure I feel growing from inside. I feel as if my hands are welded to the rock, my fingers digging into the impenetrable hardness. My body is shaking with each breath. The wind spreads my pussy lips and washes over me from anus to clit, darting into the folds of my vagina, flicking the hood of my clit, tonguing the engorged organ over and over, sucking and pulling, hungrily lapping the juices that flowed from me. My butt grounds itself into the rock, trying to push itself into the granite. Warmth spreads from inside, flowing liquid, molten, outward and up, enveloping my body. Then fire, fed by my invisible lover with its thousands of fingers and tongues, glows and builds in my pussy, down deep, at my core, grows in heat and intensity, spreading up through my stomach, enflaming my breasts, my lungs, until my breath comes in ragged gulps, building to a sobbing scream, filling me, expanding me, bursting from my body, mouth gaping, head thrown back, gasping for air, again and again and again, my body convulsing, out of control, pulsing with a heartbeat not my own. Then the aftershocks of orgasm, my pussy snapping up, clenching with uncontrollable spasms, and relaxing, falling, over and over until sobs wrack my body, a tiny voice pleading, panting, 'please ... please ... please ... please' and 'no more ... no more ...

oh God ... please ... no more,' until they become whispers lost on the breath of the wind.

Clare, 22, student

I think about this several times a month; it occurs during masturbation and sexual relations. I've had this fantasy for several years –at least five – up to now. I've never experienced it and am not sure I would want to, although I did watch one couple make love once.

When I'm having sex with my boyfriend, I sometimes imagine that we're at it in a plush hotel room: sunken bath, king-size bed and shag-pile carpet. Suddenly, the maid walks in, dressed in the clichéd tiny black skirt, white apron and blouse. But instead of apologizing, she stands and stares. My boyfriend asks her to join us. He doesn't have sex with her. She just touches us and gets touched. Then he asks her to have oral sex with me while he masturbates. I wouldn't want to do this in real life – I'm too jealous. It's just something that helps me orgasm.

Anne, 32, accountant

My husband and I were married for five years, and as for me, I considered our sex together as 'great'. It was definitely not the reason we divorced (him sleeping with my best friend was!). We did many things to make our sex interesting and not boring, like role playing, dressing up as a whore, and rape skits.

Our favourite was that I am a prostitute and the best lay in the house. I am the one always asked for by the clients. The other girls hate me because of how good I am. I still sometimes masturbate to that one, remembering how I used to tie him up and tease him for hours.

Pixie (no other information given)

Since I am bi/curious, I love fantasizing about being with a girl and my boyfriend at the same time. Having sex with him, then having her lick me out would be great, as well as putting a show on for my boyfriend. I also just love the idea of making out with another female and playing with one.

Marcia, 27, technician

Ménages à trois are a theme of my fantasies, some of which involve other women, some another woman and a man – sometimes that man is my husband, sometimes he's a stranger.

At different times, you go through different fantasies. I've had periods when I've fantasized about women a lot, and others when my fantasies were totally male – sweaty bodies, cops, and firemen.

I also regularly fantasize about having five or six sexy Adonises lining up to have sex with me. Sometimes my husband is there and watching, sometimes he even joins in and gives one of the guys a blowjob.

Another favourite is weird and wild stuff, like this one where I slather my husband in baby oil, then jump naked out of an airplane together, tied to a single parachute, so he can do me from behind.

Sean, 31, architect

A line-up of men are waiting to screw me. I lie on a mattress on the floor and the randy boys stand there with huge erections and come in me one by one. I would never want to experience this – it would make me feel cheap. But it's a sexy idea.

In another, three of us are in a room: me, a guy and a girl. They look familiar but I don't know who they are. The girl is about my height and looks a little like me. She tells me I'm pretty. We start kissing and undressing each other. The guy has a swimmer's body and sun-bleached blonde hair. He's watching from a few feet away. Soon he's joining us and we are one erotic tangle of bodies.

Patricia, 28, estate agent

I like to think of a train of young guys standing waiting to have sex with me. Each one that comes into me is so hard and excited and he thrusts and thrusts so good and is so powerful when he comes.

Another fantasy is one where I am in a place – I don't know exactly where – but everyone is running around naked and making love all the time. Men with women, women with women, men with men – it doesn't matter. What matters is pleasure.

Donna, 27, news reporter

This fantasy is based on a club a friend told me about where there is sex in the back room. In my fantasy, the club has a dark room. The concept is you enter a blacked-out room, and engage in 'anything goes' sex. You have no idea who you are with, or what they are going to do. Talking is allowed, but conversation is discouraged.

I know in real life I could never go to such a place. But in my fantasy, I dress in my sexiest outfit – a body-clinging red silk that barely skims my hips, high red stilettos and black fishnet stockings. I approach a building with one door. There is a bouncer there and I worry he is going to turn me away. But he looks me over from head to toe, grunts, and slowly swings the door open.

I step into a small entry where a young woman is seated on a stool. She removes my clothing and puts a black, silk cord around my neck, on which hangs a container of lubricant. She tells me to remember that there is no light at all in the room. Once I am in, the only way to get out is to head for a wall, and feel for the door, which has a raised design. You knock, and she would open it for you. I am a little surprised that it can't be opened from the inside, but realise why, when she turns off the light in the entry before opening the door.

When the light goes off, I feel enveloped by the blackness. No matter where you are, there is usually some light source, no matter how small ... the stars, the light from other rooms, the LCD on the VCR or clock radio. This is total blackness, nothing. The girl who had spoken to me pushs me gently through the door and recommends that I move away from the door. I hear the door swing shut.

I know nothing about the room I have entered. The floor is soft, but the covering feels more like padding than carpeting. Sounds of sex come from various parts of the room. I start to take a few steps forward and trip, falling flat on my face. Feeling around, I deduce that I have tripped on a pillow.

Deciding that hands and knees are probably more my speed, I crawl forward. I head toward a sound ... the rather wet sound of a cock sliding in and out of a pussy. The woman is moaning softly, the man breathing quite heavily. Before I get there I encounter flesh, warm and sweaty, a foot. My hands slide over a hairy leg. I continue to slide upward, cupping a pair of balls.

'Oh yeah, that feels good,' a deep voice groans.

I push his legs apart and crawl between them. My mouth makes contact ... but not with his cock. I slide my mouth over his body slowly, not wanting to lose contact in the darkness. Finally my mouth finds his cock, and I pull it into my mouth. I move my head over him, sucking him deep into my throat. My hands begin stroking his body, exploring.

I feel someone come up behind me, and a hard cock press against my back. He kneels behind me as his hands explore my body from behind, cupping my breasts, rubbing them. I lean back a little against the hard chest, letting the cock slide from my mouth.

'Oh, God, please don't stop,' he moans.

The man behind me pulls me aside and slides his mouth over the cock. The guy who I had been sucking is moaning louder now. I search for the second man's cock and stroke it slowly. The man standing up cries out when he comes, thanking me.

'My pleasure,' purrs another man.

The cock in my hand is rock hard, a drop of pre-cum oozing from the tip as my fingers slide over the head. I crawl in front of him, whispering, 'Fuck me,' on the way past.

His hands grasp my hips, pulling me toward him, spreading me wide. His cock pauses only briefly at the entrance to my cunt before driving deep within. I gasp as he begins to fuck me furiously. He pulls almost all the way out before driving deep inside again. I feel more hands sliding over me, stroking my face, then lower down my body.

A mouth fastens on my clit, pulling it into a warm, wet mouth. I scream out when my orgasm hits. The cock continues to pound in and out of me, the mouth staying locked on my clit, and juices flow freely from me. A finger slides into my anus, slowly, insistently. A second finger joins it and soon the fingers and cock are moving in unison.

I climax again.

The man fucking me orgasms, his semen dripping from my cunt when he withdraws. The mouth between my legs keeps licking it from me. The guy who has been fucking me turns me towards him and kisses me softly, his tongue pressing into my mouth.

I feel someone move behind him. I move back to 'feel' what is happening. I run my tongue along his side, meeting a face in the darkness. A quick kiss is exchanged. I move forward, my face brushing the other ... soft skin. I explore her body, lingering on her breasts, which are big and round, with rock-hard nipples.

I guide the cock of the guy we are caressing to her vagina. I slide one finger into her hole slowly, moving it around, savouring the juiciness. She moans, but doesn't pull away, so I add a second finger, wiggling them slightly. I use my second hand to explore her clit.

I free both hands and grasp the nearby cock, bringing him closer to the woman kneeling on the floor. I spread her lips wide apart while the long, thick cock slides into her. Her moans increase, not begging to stop, but begging to go on.

I can feel the movement as the man begins to fuck her.

Meanwhile, I feel a tongue licking between my legs. I slide to the floor, letting the sensations wash over me, eventually reaching another climax.

I continue my crawl across the floor. I am exhausted. I need to find the door and get out. As I leave, I hear behind me the grunts and moans of people being satisfied.

Dorothy

I stand at the kitchen counter with my back to you. We've finished eating dinner hours ago, and I've been chopping vegetables for tomorrow night's salad. You walk up behind me, and your big, warm hands slide around my waist and under the edge of my top. Your fingers press firmly across my tummy, meeting just over my belly button, as you bend to give my neck an open mouthed kiss and slowly nibble up my neck.

'Mmmmm, keep that up and I'll never get this finished,' I whisper in your ear as I lean my head back against your shoulder and give your earlobe a quick nibble. I begin to slowly stir the salad with a big fork. The noodles slip and slide, and all the tiny bits of onion, green pepper and tomato fall down over the sides, landing in the bottom of the bowl.

I raise my head again and continue with my work, but my efforts now seem fruitless. You chuckle. Then you dig your hand deep into the bowl and begin to mix the whole mess. I reach into the bowl, snatching a cluster of noodles and tomato bits between my fingertips, and raise them high above your head so you can catch the tail end on the tip of your tongue. Then I slowly lower it in a spiral motion, coiling it onto the surface of your tongue. 'Yummmm,' you say.

I wait for you to swallow your mouthful and slide my fingers into your mouth, one by one, for you to lick and suck the oily mixture off. I lie back against your shoulder again, closing my eyes and letting myself experience the wet heat of your tongue along the surface of my fingers.

'Mmmmm, that feels good,' I murmur.

'Mmmm, that tastes good,' you counter.

I smile in answer and your mouth lowers over mine. You reach into the bowl, take the end of a stray noodle, and raise your mouth from mine, trailing it across my lips. The oil drips across my chin. Your tongue quickly laps it up and continues along my lips, slurping the noodles in as you go.

Scooping a modest handful up, you bring it over my cleavage and let the noodles slip over the edge of your palm, plopping a few at a time, down the front of my low cut top; then you lower your hand to rub the greasy mess in.

I let my head fall back with a thump and begin to giggle. The cold noodles feel good against the top of my breasts, and I feel the oil dribble down between them.

You turn me to face you now and bend to grab the stray noodles clinging to my skin using your tongue and teeth. It feels so good. The contrast of cold pasta and warm tongue sends shivers up my spine, and my body arches against yours. I reach back, grabbing a large handful without you realizing it, and quickly grab your belt, giving it a little tug and dumping the cold, slippery salad down the front of your shorts. You let out a loud yelp and my hands immediately begin to rub you through the material there.

You squirm under my hands. 'This is my favourite way to eat pasta,' I say, looking up into your eyes. I hold your gaze as I slowly lower myself to my knees in front of you, pulling your fly down as I go. Your eyes get bigger as you anticipate what I'm about to do.

I feel your member poking outward at me, begging for my attention, and I open your pants. Spaghetti hangs from your shaft, like tinsel on a Christmas tree, and I smile and look forward to the feast I'm about to enjoy. My tongue reaches out and wraps around the end of one of the long noodles and I slowly suck it into my mouth. The slippery spaghetti slides across your erect member and disappears between my moist lips. You moan at the sight, wishing it was you being sucked into my mouth instead. Shivers tingle up and down your spine as I do it again and again, and you hear the slurping, smacking, sucking noises so close to your anxious flesh. You lean back against the side counter and close your eyes.

I wrap my greasy lips around your member, sucking you deep into my warm mouth and sliding my tongue around you over and over. You let a deep, growling moan escape your lips and push your hips towards me. My hands cup your tensing cheeks and pull you in as far as I can. I moan loud and long, sending vibrations up into your groin, already alive with delightful sensations.

Your body quivers, and I feel you growing tenser with each thrust. I squeeze you gently with my tongue, moaning over and over, creating a wave-like effect.

Your knees grow weak, and you hold onto the counter and let the feelings engulf you until your body allows you to release. I feel your cheeks tense hard, and your whole body begins to spasm as I feel your warm fluids against the back of my throat. I swallow all you have to offer, and when you begin to relax again I let you slowly slide off my tongue.

I return to my feet, kissing your chest as I open the buttons on your shirt. My hands caress you, and I find your hardened nipples one by one, giving each a little attention.

You peel my clingy top away from my breasts and off my shoulders, letting it fall to the floor. Then you reach around and unhook my lacy bra and let it follow suit. Your hands feel wonderful slipping across my breasts, rubbing the oil into my skin. You reach down from time to time with your eager tongue and lick the dressing that clings to my skin.

My breasts are covered with goose bumps as my mind tries to decipher this spontaneous sensual outburst of yours. I've known you to be playful at times, but never quite like this.

You pull me into your arms, my pelvis against yours, warm through my remaining clothing. I feel your hard shaft against me and reach down to unfasten my jeans and slide my panties downward, allowing it contact with my warm body.

Your hands seek out the warmth within, and it's not long before your fingers find my moist, hot centre. I gasp at the swiftness of your oil slick digits, and my back curls in response. I let out a long, low moan, almost like a soft purring, and you work my flesh with an expertise almost unfamiliar to me.

There's a fire within you tonight I've never seen. I feel an urgency, and it ignites my passion further, bringing the flame to a white hot glow. You push my jeans down over my hips with your unoccupied hand and bend down on one knee to reach down and pull them off, one leg at a time, my panties following close behind. I feel your warm breath tickle across my naked mound and feel your tongue sneak a sample taste. My hands begin to gently play with your hair as my hips begin to move in rhythm against your face. I lean the small of my back against the counter as you grasp my firm derrière and plunge your tongue deeper, spreading my legs a little wider with your hungry mouth.

You moan and growl with passion unleashed, breathing in my musky scent. Your passion seems to feed on itself, and I quickly reach a tactile summit. I feel your tongue rubbing against my most sensitive spots and driving me into a sexual frenzy. My knees grow weak over and over until I think I might collapse altogether. Your tongue flicks harder and harder over my aroused flesh, and I soon feel the warmth begin to spread from my centre, upward and outward, to all my extremities, bathing me in a kind of warm glowing awareness. I feel my pelvic muscles contract and expand with intense pleasure around your still active tongue.

You moan at the sweet taste of my nectar as it moistens your face and dribbles down your chin, and you press me closer still, not wanting to waste one precious drop. My body is exhausted and I cling to the counter for support. You lower me to the floor then and caress my breasts gently with your open hand.

When my breathing returns to a normal pace you begin to play with my nipple, using your tongue. It doesn't take long before I am turned on once again. You kiss up and down my body and I pull you to me with my hands. Your knees straddle me and I coax you upward, over my body until your hips are over my ribcage. Your hard member slides between my ample breasts in a rhythmic rocking motion. I feel you grow slick and slippery and I long to taste you. I reach out with my tongue to touch your tip as you slide through and you slow your pace, wanting more contact.

I purse my lips and let your head slide between them and into the moist heat of my hungry mouth. 'Mmmmmm, you feel so smooth on my tongue. Like liquid velvet.'

You become more and more urgent and, raising yourself up, drive your slick firmness deep into my throat. I yield to you, sucking gently, then firmer in rhythm with your body. I feel you throbbing and pulsing against my hot tongue, longing for release. I long for it too.

You continue until I feel your cheeks go rigid and then I intensify my grasp on you and pull you into a higher orgasmic state. You howl out loud, like a wounded animal, and let the sensations engulf you. I feel your leg muscles quiver and watch your face as your creamy liquid lust shoots against the back of my palate. I swallow in great gulps. You have a look of peaceful bliss on your face.

Rose, 34, banker

I've always wanted to have a threesome. A guy and a girl. I'd like to suck off the guy as the girl sucks me off ... also I would like to jerk him off all over the girl and then lick it off her tits. I masturbate regularly to this fantasy. In fact, I am getting hot now thinking about doing it and watching the girl's face.

I also love the thought of having two guys at once, but not just with all their attention focused on me, I want to see them really get off on touching and licking and fucking each other too ... that's my hottest fantasy ... each person really turned on by the other two ... The possibilities are endless!!!

I'm going to have to go off and think about all this now!!! In depth!

Celia, 32, senior brand manager

I love imagining a guy fucking me while in turn another guy was fucking him! Just think of the force pounding into me!

Yum!! Just thinking about it is a huge turn-on ... I'd also love to have two guys in my mouth at the same time (although I'm not sure how I'd manage!), their cocks rubbing against each other and my tongue! Makes me sopping wet just thinking about it!

Another thing I fantasize about is having one guy fuck me in my puss and another in my ass. WOW! That would be amazing! And knowing that they could feel each other through my membrane and getting off even more because of it ...

I love the thought of that kind of closeness, the guys' balls banging together as they fuck me senseless, their cocks rubbing against each other through the thin wall inside me ... I want them to really get off on each other as well as me!!

Dot, 28, salesperson

One of my BIGGEST fantasies is being with two women, fucking one with a vibrator, and having the other fuck me in the ass with a strap-on.

Another secret fantasy of mine is to have two men to satisfy my every whim! I'd tell them both just what to do to pleasure me for hours, making me come again and again ... and then when I'd had my fill of them and couldn't possibly take any more, I'd instruct them to suck and fuck each other for my viewing pleasure ... even if they didn't want to, I'd make them, and they would both enjoy all of it so much!

It's strange for me to have this kind of fantasy, because I always want to give as much as I get ... but it IS a good fantasy! It gets me very hot and wet!

Ellen, 28, publisher

I love fantasizing about being with two guys. The thought of one guy licking my clit while the other's cock is in my wet pussy ... oh my! I could cum now thinking about it. I like the thought of getting all that attention to myself (because, of course, it's MY fantasy and therefore, I would be the object of adoration!) Sometimes, I fantasize about one man in my mouth and the other buried deep in the other end. I really can't imagine how that would be – probably not all that great in reality – but it makes a hell of a sexy fantasy.

forbidden
thrills

Introduction

All fantasies are basically a risk-free arena to explore all your deepest, most prurient sexual interests without moral, legal, or physical consequences. None do so much as the so-called forbidden fantasies – erotic daydreams about sex with your father or brother, a young neighbourhood boy, someone who is a different race or even a favoured pet.

There are a few different explanations for these illicit fantasies. For instance, there's some speculation that imagining having sex with a family member is less about the actual pleasure and more about healing a relationship with someone close to you. This may be a comment on your connection with the actual person you are fantasizing about or they may be a stand-in for someone else close to you. Through the fantasy, you create a sense of intimacy that you feel may be missing in reality.

Meanwhile, imagining yourself as a teacher in sex is a way of taking control. Just as men treasure the virginal maiden fantasy, for many women, there is a special thrill in taking part in a man's first sexual experience. Some experts say it may also be a way of reliving your own sexual deflowering in a more positive light.

Sex with someone who is of a different skin colour than you is also about control. Often, different races are associated with different sexual myths – Asians are skilled in the mysterious erotic aspects of lovemaking, black men are well-endowed, Jewish men are thought to be especially caring and so on. Fantasies about these men puts you in control of their so-called strangeness, letting you experience something different without danger.

Some women fantasize about having sex with or in the presence of an animal. It is almost as if animals – and the naturalness of sex to them – enhance the sexual excitement a person may feel. Dogs tend to be more common than cats – possibly because cats aren't lickers like dogs. Horses are also popular – one theory is that these women may have ridden when growing up and had their first orgasm literally in the saddle. Also, the sheer size of a horse's sexual organs are so obvious and sexual that they become a visual turn-on that practically demands fantasy. It's unlikely anyone really wants to be fucked by something the size of a cricket bat – but as a fantasy, it's highly exciting to imagine oneself being so utterly filled.

The bottom line, though, is that all of these fantasies are exciting because of their taboo quality. Let's face it, without the hint of the forbidden, no sex – whether it crosses social lines or not – would seem quite so naughty. And if you are fantasizing about sex with your father or pet dog, then anything becomes possible – like unlimited orgasms or being perceived as the most desirable woman in the world.

Gabrielle, 26, gym instructor

I sometimes masturbate to the fantasy of having a young man about 15. He comes to visit for some reason and is very attractive and sexy – a young Liam Neeson – but a bit shy. I can tell he's attracted to me, but he's a virgin and doesn't know what to do. We talk for a long time. We're sitting and we keep moving closer and closer to each other. Finally, I take his hand. Slowly, tenderly, I seduce him. We lie down. I undress him slowly, touching his body all over as I undress for him. We make beautiful love, over and over again.

Another fantasy I have is that I am lying on a mattress naked. On top of me is an old boyfriend, but as a young boy. He has lots of new curly hair on his chest and he is very slippery, especially down below. My muscles tense and we come.

Nichola, 30, nanny

When I was younger, I didn't have particular fantasies, only being with someone older and more experienced. These days, I think about seducing a younger man! Let me tell you my favourite fantasy.

This fantasy is based on a real incident with a 13 year-old boy. I was 25 at the time. I was working as a playground assistant and this kid used to bring his little brother and hang around. He was just entering puberty and his body was half-way between being a man and still a boy. All summer, we flirted with 'accidental' touching. Finally one day we played hide-and-seek with all the kids and found ourselves behind some bushes. We kissed and held each other. That's all that happened, but I fantasize about this untouched male virgin having his first sexual encounter with me. He lays me down on a bench, lies on top of me, takes out his throbbing, perfect penis and begs me to let him in. I always masturbate to climax thinking about it.

Carla, 31, marketing manager

I have had fantasies about sleeping with a younger man for a while. It has nothing to do with my love for my husband. This is carnal. Animalistic. Exciting. One of my favourites involves a young man who sometimes comes to the bank where I work to do business.

I imagine that we have made a rendezvous at a local hotel where he works. I get there late and am directed to go down a long hallway and to knock on an office door. When I open the door, I see him, on the telephone, his long legs resting on top of the desk in front of him.

Although I know that he is 6ft 4in, his size overwhelms me. But what are more amazing are his eyes. Steve has the most beautiful blue eyes I have ever seen. They are clear blue, like the sky, and they sparkle with his smile. Finally, he hangs up the telephone.

I stand there frozen, with my overnight case in my hand. He walks over to me and gently takes the suitcase out of my hand and places it against the wall. In the same swift movement, he walks over to the door of the office and dead-bolts it.

The knot in my stomach returns as he takes my hand and leads me over to the swivel chair behind the desk. He sits down and places me on his lap. Reaching up with both hands he takes my face and gently kisses my lips. His lips are warm and full of the heat that is inside both of us.

The kiss becomes passionate as his tongue probes my mouth, searching for a deeper intensity. His strong arms are behind my back, pulling me closer to his chest and the embrace is so tight that for a moment I can barely breathe.

I push him away to study his face. He has strong cheekbones and a beautiful nose and he smells of flour and sugar, almost like a baked sugar cookie. I smile. He is just as beautiful as I had expected and all I want to do is to make endless love to him in the middle of the office, in the middle of the day. But I feel funny because of our age differences.

I break the silence, 'Steve ...' I say, my voice surprisingly cracking with an emotion I do not know I have.

He puts his fingers on my lips and smiles, as if he knows what I was going to say.

'Don't speak. I like older women, I find them attractive, I find them sexy, I find them wonderful.'

'How old are you anyway?' I ask.

'I'm 24.' He kisses me again. 'I have been waiting for this for so long. Just let me lead, and just follow. You are so beautiful in person. You are such a woman. Just let me have you.' His voice is hoarse with his need.

He slowly starts unbuttoning my blouse, kissing my neck, and making his way down to my breasts. He gently takes one of my breasts in his hand and kisses my nipple. The sensation sends immediate wetness to my pussy and I feel as though I am going to climax right there in his lap.

As he continues to unbutton my blouse, I feel his hot tongue running down my belly to the top of my slacks. He shifts my body so that my head is resting on the desk, as he unzips my slacks and unbuckles my belt.

The fear of someone walking in is not only more erotic to me but also exciting and dangerous and my whole body starts to quiver. I feel his cock growing harder beneath my spine and the feeling shows me that he is as big as he looked like he was going to be. But he does not stop there. He gently lifts my hips and begins to pull my slacks off my body, all the while giving me deep kisses, wonderful kisses that go right inside my soul.

In a swift motion, he lifts my body and places me on the desk. He pushes everything on the desk to the floor with a crashing sound and starts laughing. I laugh too, feeling like I am in some sort of movie.

Steve continues to remove my slacks and my panties in one swift motion that only an experienced lover could know how to do.

I lose myself in the continual orgasms I am experiencing as his tongue probes deeper into my pussy. He spreads apart my thin outer lips and lightly flicks his tongue across my inner lips sending a sensation that wracks my body with quivering spasms of ecstasy. He buries his tongue deeper inside me, moving it back and forth at first and then, resting his chin, begins licking and eating me all over. Each time I come, I hear his breathing intensify.

And then in the same swift motion he made earlier, he rolls me over on top of him, placing me so that my pussy is over his mouth. My juices begin to fill up his mouth as he moans quietly. My hands move down to his swollen cock that is pushing up against the zipper of his pants.

I remove myself from his face and start unbuttoning his shirt, my fingers moving swiftly to his zipper since I cannot wait to have him inside my mouth. Sliding myself down his body, I place his cock deep inside my mouth, sucking on him until I feel his body arch and quiver. Small spurts of semen appear on top of his cock and I lick them off.

'Mmmm, this is so good. You're so good,' he says softly as he plays with my hair. I nuzzle my head in his balls and lick each one until I feel him jerking about ready to climax.

I want him to climax, but I want him inside me more. I climb on top of him and feel him deep inside me. He is so large that he fills me up and I feel his hardness right up to my belly button. He takes both of his hands and holds my breasts as I ride him. I bend down and kiss his beautiful mouth, his eyes, his cheekbones, praying that he will climax so that we can continue to make love with the intensity we started with.

After a few minutes, Steve rolls me over so that he is on top. His strength and his size are overwhelming to my 5ft 3in body and he places my legs on his shoulders. Feeling his cock pushing up against my clit makes me come once more and it is with that heat that I feel him come.

I kiss him again, gently. 'You smell like a cookie.' I say.

'So I've been told', he smiles. 'And now, it's time to clean the cookie up.' He lifts himself up off me and walks over to the sink in the office. He returns with a damp, warm, cloth and begins cleaning me. So gentle are his movements that it brings tears to my eyes and I touch his hand.

He leans over and kisses me on the forehead, takes a deep breath and says in a whisper, 'So ... what is it like fucking a younger man? Was it good?'

'Good? It was unbelievable,' I utter. 'I never would have believed it to be so gentle, so good.' I push back the one lock of hair that has fallen on his forehead. 'And, I want to do it again and again and again. Thank you for taking me to places I haven't been.'

Melissa, 29, restaurant manager

I fantasize a few times a week. The fantasies depend on my mood and if I'm with my partner. I normally have this fantasy when I'm trying to get to sleep at night. It relaxes me.

I am taking care of my friend's house while she is away. One day, as I stop by to pick up the post, I see a young man outside cutting the lawn. I stop a moment and watch him work. It's late in the day but still pretty hot, and he's removed his shirt. His muscles flex as he pushes the mower back and forth.

I grab a couple of beers and ask him if he wants one. As we sit on the patio drinking, I find out his name is Richard and that he's 15. I shiver looking at the slight sheen of sweat on his skin. A trickle runs down his chest and I wish I could follow it down with my tongue. I can't help but wonder exactly how wonderful he would look without his shorts as well. He is just over six feet tall, with brown hair and the most incredible blue eyes I have ever seen.

I mention how hot it is and run the bottle over my throat, feeling the cold against my warm skin.

'Does that really work?' he asks.

It's the opening I've been waiting for. I move closer to him, and slide my beer bottle over his hard chest and his upper arms. He groans in pleasure, so I slide it lower. He looks startled and slightly scared, so I kiss him and tell him I am going to make him feel wonderful. Our mouths meet, hesitantly at first, but quickly become more frantic. I can feel his erection poking into my belly and caressing it through his shorts, I ask him if he's ever had a blowjob before. He shakes his head no and mumbles that no girl has ever touched him there before. He practically jumps off the chair as I pop him out of his shorts and start licking him. He comes within seconds, holding my head tight to him. I feel incredible power as I suck him dry, knowing that I have given him his first real orgasm.

Annette, 31, editor

I often fantasize about a young man when I can't get to sleep at night. He's younger than me, but not too young. His erection is making his trousers bulge.

'Looks like you're going to have to do something about that,' I say, releasing him. He gives a small groan as I move my hands over his hard shaft. I feel in total control.

I push his head down, pressing his face deep into my wetness. I can feel his tongue probing deep within me. He spreads my legs wide and traces a path back between my legs, licking me everywhere.

My climax hits fast, my juices running down my legs. I push him back and kneel beside him, kissing him. I start at his forehead, then move down his face, which is wet with my juices. I begin to lick him lightly, my tongue just flicking against the line of his throat. Working my way slowly downward I lick his nipples, pulling each into my mouth, holding it for a few seconds.

He tries to push me further down, but I resist. This is my show and I set the pace. Sliding lower over his belly, I finally reach my goal. I pull his throbbing cock into my mouth, feeling the blood pound in it. I engulf him completely, feeling him slide deep into my throat. I begin to pump my mouth over him, using my fingers to stroke his balls and the shaft when it isn't in my mouth.

As I feel his orgasm approaching, I use my hands to lightly stroke his body as much as I can reach. His muscles tighten and he explodes, his hot seed pouring into my mouth. I swallow it all, feeling it running down my throat.

We hold each other for a while, kissing, touching, resting ... perhaps for a little more?

Georgia, 29, financial advisor

Since my early teens, my big fantasy has been to touch myself while imagining being a baby and being fondled and caressed and held by a big strong man who looked like – but wasn't – my father.

He is very loving and caring of me, making sure I feel pleasure and taking care so that his sperm doesn't go inside of me and make me pregnant.

Afterwards, he carries me to a warm bath and sponges me clean. Then he tucks me into a big soft bed with clean crisp white sheets and strokes my head until I fall asleep.

Brittany, 32, advertising director

Sometimes I fantasize about the first time I had sex, when I was 14 – but instead of my boyfriend, I imagine the guy I am with is my father or my older brother. He is much more sensuous than my boyfriend was. At the time, the whole thing was over in a minute and all I remember feeling was pain. But in my fantasy, the man focuses on my clitoris and teaches me how to caress myself. He shows me how pleasurable it is to have my nipples stroked and finds a secret place around my bum-hole that makes me moan out loud with pleasure when it is tickled. He keeps nuzzling and probing me until I am literally dripping wet and begging him to take me.

Afterwards, he shows me how to go down on a guy and give him pleasure. We continue with our 'lessons' until I am extremely skilled at receiving and giving pleasure. Then he leaves.

Anonymous

I often fantasize about being made love to by my father. In reality, he was a very remote man, but in my fantasies, he is very loving and adores me.

I am around 10. I finish my shower and turn to come out when my daddy enters the room with a towel. I am surprised as I am obviously too old to be dried and dressed. I feel funny, but it's my dad, so I start towel drying my hair while he watches. I move down to my body, but he says, 'Let me do it.'

He rubs my body until it tingles and is rosy pink. Then he takes my hand and leads me into the bedroom where my nightie is laid on the bed waiting for me. I reach up to give him a hug and thank him for his caring help. He turns his face so my kiss lands on his lips. The kiss deepens. It is frightening but strangely alluring at the same time. I pull back and he seems to understand what I am feeling because he offers to rub baby powder into my skin. 'But Daddy, I'm not a baby!' I giggle. But he tells me it will make me feel good and dry all over, so I say okay.

SEX FANTASIES BY WOMEN FOR WOMEN

He tells me to lay on my stomach, so I lay down on my bed, at first unsure but after a while it feels so nice that I start to relax. After all, this is my daddy, he wouldn't hurt me. His hands start to wander down my back and over my legs and he playfully spanks my behind. When I start to protest, he says that it's okay, reminding me that this is a game we used to play when I was a little girl.

But then he spanks me again a little harder. I try to escape. He spanks me again, not so hard this time. Then his spanking turns into something else. 'Mmmm, that feels good,' I moan, not even realizing I am speaking out loud. 'Daddy, more please, more please ... ooohhh!' He has reached down and started licking me between my legs.

I am yearning for what only he can give me. I squirm with the feelings he is causing inside of me. I am getting warm and wet. I want more.

Then all of a sudden he is turning me over. Oh God! His tongue keeps on licking and torturing me. It is running over and over my warm, wet pussy. His hands are squeezing my young breasts. He is squeezing them and pinching them with his fingertips. I am going wild with wanting him. His fingers replace his tongue between my legs. I am being driven wild with hunger.

Is this right? I wonder. Does every little girl feel this way when her father touches her? He tells me it will be our special loving. He tells me he wants to kiss me. 'Let me kiss you, baby. Daddy wants to show you how much he loves his little girl.'

'I love you too, Daddy,' I moan as he presses his fingers into me. He puts his arms around me and pulls me close so I can feel his hard body against mine. His penis is poking into my tummy. I beg him to put it in me.

'Baby, are you ready for me?' he asks. 'I don't want to hurt you.' He slips inside of me and since I am a virgin, it does hurt a little, but he tells me how much he loves me and the pain melts into something else as he starts moving against me. It feels good but so big. He seems pleased when I start pushing my hips with him. 'That's it, baby girl,' he encourages. We rock together like our bodies were made for each other. We move faster and faster until we finally come, feelings so good and warm and close. I know no one else has ever made him feel so good.

Tina, 27, recruitment officer

I made up this fantasy when I was on holiday with my boyfriend. There was a black man who was at the hotel and I obsessed about him constantly. Maybe his dark skin made him more exotic, I'm not sure. But I wanted this man.

I imagine myself wearing just a bikini and bumping into him near the pool. Instead of apologizing, I kiss him hard. He kisses back just as much. His fingers pull my bikini top off and he tells me how beautiful I am.

His mouth leaves mine and he begins to kiss my body. He licks and kisses my nipples, sending shivers through me. I can't remember when he gets undressed, but somehow he is naked, and beautiful in his own way. His dark skin glistens, it has such depth to it. I lean forward and kiss his shoulder, wondering if he tastes any different than my boyfriend. Oh, and he does ... so musky, so sweet. Hard to describe, but so different.

He pushes me back on the pool deck and slips off my bikini bottoms. He moves down between my legs. I can see my barely tanned legs on his dark shoulders. I am so busy marvelling at the differences between us that it is a shock when his mouth comes down on me. I feel his tongue licking between my legs and I can't believe it. His fingers slide over my pubic hair, tracing patterns. His teeth nip lightly before his tongue probes inside of me.

I can feel myself reacting instinctively as I push forward against him. I cry out in disappointment as his tongue leaves me, but gasp in pleasure as his fingers take over. I lose the struggle to keep him to me as my legs slide off his shoulders. He leans over me, mouth going back to exploring my body. Fingers plunge in and out of my cunt rapidly, driving me wild. I can't believe how my body is responding to this stranger. I can even feel his cock brushing against my leg now as I come closer to my climax.

I pull him to me with my arms as I begin to feel the flood overtaking my body. I want to feel him against me as I cry out. My wet come coats his fingers, still pressed deep inside of me. He is hard now, oh, so hard. He moves forward and his cock brushes the wetness between my thighs. I push him away though, there is something I want to do first.

I can hear my own voice, strong and filled with lust, 'No, I want to feel your cock in my mouth first.'

Though the voice is mine, the words are ones I never use. I start to kneel, but he stops me. He moves us both onto a deck chair and slowly moves around, so his erect cock is brushing my cheek.

I move my head slightly, capturing him in my mouth. As his cock slides deeper into my mouth, I can feel the throb of it inside of me. I pull my head back and let him slide out, so I can explore him more. My tongue traces a path down the shaft, following a pulsing vein. He is definitely thicker than my boyfriend is, but about the same length. The colour is so different though, so dark, the head a purple black, the shaft a dark chocolate shade.

He tries to guide my head back to the tip of his cock, but I'm not ready yet. I begin licking and kissing him slowly. I am in control. His hands relax and he lets me set the pace. I can't get over the feel of his cock. I let it rub slowly over my cheek. I feel like it could last forever. But that isn't fair to him. I move slightly and capture the tip of his cock between my lips. I push forward, feeling him slide in gradually. I haven't opened my mouth wide enough and my teeth rake lightly along his shaft.

My hands explore his dark skin as my mouth moves over his rock hard shaft. His hands wrap around my head, his cock now pumping in and out of my mouth. Suddenly, though, his warm come fills my mouth.

I come at the same time.

Lee, 28, credit controller

I don't have fantasies during sex. On rare occasions, my partner and I will create one together, usually a seductive one that we act out. However, once we start to have intercourse with each other, I become involved with the sensations and what he and I are doing to each other.

But fantasies really come in when I masturbate. They are usually a variation on this one: I am with an Indian man. I am his willing slave. He has a very long thin penis which seems to be able to bend and can caress every inch of my vagina – it even manages to press against my clitoris while it is inside of me. My lover whispers in my ear that in order to have good karma, we must do every position in the Kama Sutra. We spend the rest of our lives locked together in sexual ecstasy.

Linda, 25, merchandiser

When I was about 14, I developed an obsession with black men. It had nothing to do with being racist. Something to do with Denzel Washington, I think, whom I think is one of the sexiest men alive. In this fantasy, I am at a party, getting a drink from the kitchen. I am a little drunk and flirting with this black man who has been chatting me up all night. I guess in real life, people would be coming in and out, but this is my fantasy, so we are suddenly all alone.

Suddenly, he starts kissing me. I have always been curious what it would be like to make love to someone who is a different race than me (I'm white). He leans me against the counter, sliding to the floor between my legs. He pushes aside my panties and his tongue quickly finds my clitoris. His fingers hold me open and his tongue flicks against my nub. I stagger a little as I come, juices flowing from my cunt.

He stands back up and kisses my breast, taking the nipple into his mouth. I look down and see his dark face outlined against my white breast and it makes me hot. He bites my nipple softly, then moves upward, his mouth sliding over my neck and face, then softly nipping my ear. He turns me around, leaning me against the counter. He spreads my legs and slides his cock into me quickly. I gasp a little at its size, which is long and thick.

This is a fast and furious fuck, no holds barred. By the time we have both climaxed we are out of breath. We adjust our clothing and return to the party.

Vanessa, 25, waitress

I have a natural attraction for white men (I'm West Indian). I know that my family would disown me if I ever ended up with a white guy, but they are the ones I fantasize about. I like to think about my dark skin contrasted against a really white chest. All I have to do is picture his white cock sliding in and out of my hot, juicy, dark vagina to come.

Jenna, 28, violinist

I like to think of a black man standing next to my bed. I don't know who he is or how he has gotten in. He is naked and his penis is unbelievably large – at least 10 inches – and standing high. Then he touches himself and asks if I want some. His body is dark and shining with sweat. He is beautiful and even though I know it is dangerous, I also know that I must have him. He fills me until I am almost in pain. When he comes, it's so strong I feel like I am being caught in a wave of ecstasy.

Anonymous

It turns me on when our golden retriever Simma is in the room when I have sex. I sometimes fantasize he is there even when he isn't. I like to think he is getting erect listening to us. Sometimes, I imagine he joins in, licking us and taking me from behind while my boyfriend screws me from the front.

Antonia, 26, potter

I grew up on a farm, so I saw lots of animals copulating from a young age, which turned me on. Around 13, I started fantasizing about doing it with a dog or a horse. I still have these fantasies now. The weird thing is, I don't fantasize about my own dog – I fantasize about a neighbour's dog – as if doing it with my own dog would be incest!

Another fantasy I have are scenes on the beach or in a grassy meadow surrounded by heavy, dark forests, I am nude, usually running in the wind with another person. He is tall, strong and very tanned – not in that playboy sunbathing way, but in a rugged, outdoors way. There is usually a dapple grey horse with us that may be grazing – or we play and ride it. We have sex on the horse. Me in front of him, while he plays with my breasts. The movement of the horse pushes us over the edge. We then sleep and the horse keeps watch nearby.

Sarah, 24, stock controller

In all my sexual fantasies, I am always dressed in soft sensuous clothes, very revealing – the colours are always dark or black. There is always a female dog somewhere around with whom I am in complete accord or communication – it is almost as if she is me, but an animal.

In these fantasies, I am very attractive to many men, but they cannot reach me. They want to get to me, but the dog keeps them away. Then the dog starts to lick me slowly and lovingly until I orgasm.

Tricia, 28, consultant

Sometimes I have had a dog come and sniff and lick my cunt. It was exciting and I get very sexy thinking about it. Also, I get off thinking about a German Shepherd or Doberman fucking me. One time the German Shepherd down the street came into my house. He used to visit me a lot, but this one time I must have been ovulating or something because he kept trying to jump up on me to have sex. I finally made him leave. But I sure fantasize about letting him fuck me. His name was Oliver. Sometimes I used a vibrator to masturbate and pretend that it's Oliver fucking me.

Beth, 27, public relations officer

I have a fantasy about my friend's large shaggy dog Rex (the funny thing is I have always kidded my friend that her dog's name sounds like a porn star name!) My friend asks me to live in her apartment while she is abroad and care for Rex. At bedtime, he becomes very playful and increasingly sexually aggressive – both with his tongue and his penis – until he finally has me across the bed, at which point he fucks me. I know he has done this with my girlfriend – she told me how wild it was – and I think it might be sexy to try one day.

Tania, 25, musician

My fantasy is based on something that happened when I was 15 and we were moving to another area in the city. I said I would stay at the old house for the night while everyone else stayed at the new place. It was cold and snowy out and I saw a red labrador outside running the neighbourhood. He looked so cold I invited him in. I gave him some food and he was really friendly. I petted him and slowly put my hand on his sheath. It was already getting hard. It really turned me on. I had never touched a real cock. Nothing happened, but this is the fantasy I have now:

In reality, I turfed the dog out. In my fantasy I take off my clothes. He seems excited to see me like this. He starts licking my cunt and my asshole. It feels so good, I love it. It is making me moan and I am in heaven.

I get him to lie down and I touch his cock some more and it gets real big and hard. There is a knot at the base and it is so big. I have never seen a dog's penis and it excites me. It comes out of its sheath and is skinny and pink and pointed. It is different to a guy's penis. I think since he has licked me, why not? So I lick his penis. It makes me so hot I almost come. He enjoys it too, and starts squirting some semen into my mouth. I swallow it all. It tastes so good. God, this dog is turning me on.

I stop sucking him and continue stroking him. I get up on all fours and he gets up. He licks my asshole some more, really turning me on. I start stroking his penis and he starts humping and then without warning he jumps onto my back. He is trying desperately to fuck me but is jabbing me with his penis. I reach under me to guide it into me. It doesn't take much and when he finds the mark he starts fucking me like a madman. It is so animalistic, and wild, I love it. It feels so good sliding into me and feeling his fur on my back. This has to be the ultimate experience.

We both come and then, just like I've seen dogs in real life when they are fucking, I imagine he has become stuck in me. We have to lie there so I start up again. This goes on and on until I masturbate myself to exhaustion.

Rose, 29, housewife

I have lots of fantasies, but they are all based on something that happened when I was a teenager. During that summer break on my 14th birthday, my cousin Julie and I spent a lot of time together. We slept over at each other's houses every weekend and almost every other day. I was sort of naive I guess and so was she. We were both virgins but of course we always had boys on our minds.

On one such night, hotter than hell we were camped out on the floor in sleeping bags in her room watching television and eating junk. On some of the prior nights that she or I had slept over, we had gotten into my daddy's booze cabinet and this night, we were drinking some of my uncle's beer. As usual we started talking about the guys at school and girl stuff when she said that her brother was away for the weekend and that he had some real cool sex books. She hurried to get them and we giggled and started looking at them. We posed and pretended that we were the models. It was funny but after awhile I jumped back under my sleeping bag and she into hers. We still looked at the mags and exchanged them, he must have had around 20 of them.

We giggled at some of the girl-on-girl ones and we wondered how such big dicks could go into little holes without hurting. I began to touch myself commenting how horny I was, I couldn't help it. Maybe the booze was in effect and Julie was touching herself as well under her sleeping bag while we looked at the mags. We were getting very excited and we mutually masturbated until we came. Before then, we never talked about playing with ourselves but it was obvious that we both had been doing it for some time. Now we were doing it together, it was a real turn-on.

I felt a little guilty and regretful the next morning but by Monday, I was over it. The following Wednesday I slept over at her house again and of course it didn't take long for us to sneak some mags out to look at. I was hoping we would and I think she did too. We played with ourselves again that night and we even touched each other's boobs to compare to see whose were harder.

Neither of us had the nerve to make the first move, although now of course I knew she was thinking the same thing. I think I always did have a little crush on her ... her beautiful long brown hair and nice shape, I wanted to look more like her but never really thought of her in that way.

Suddenly, while we were playing around, her dog got up from his mat in the corner and started to bark. Her dog is a German Shepherd and he was always in the room with us as usual, but this time we were nude. Cocoa started sniffing around and Julie put her muff right in his face. To her surprise, he darted his tongue out at it and licked it! This startled Julie and she jumped. We looked at each other and laughed.

We said, 'Let's try to get Cocoa to lick us!' Needless to say I was very horny at the thought and also a little scared. We tried and tried but it seemed like Cocoa wasn't going to do it. Julie even tried to play with his little dick but no action. Cocoa would not play. But we started talking about how dogs and animals do it and we just got hornier and hornier. We masturbated ourselves until we came and we went to sleep.

Over the years, all my fantasies have always been about being licked and fucked by a dog.

the
male mind

Introduction

Erotic fantasies provide a unique insight into the different scripts that may underlie sexual behaviour in men and women. Men's fantasies reflect basic male instincts. One study estimates that men mate in their mind an average of seven times a day. That's 2,555 times a year. Another study found that more than half of all men spend 10 per cent of their time in sexual la-la land. In fact, men spend far more time daydreaming about sex than they do actually having it. Even Hefner. Even Beatty. Even men who are on their honeymoons.

The main item on the agenda is sheer lust and physical gratification. There are rarely encumbering relationships, emotional elaboration, complicated plot lines, flirtation, courtship and extended foreplay. Rather, the main focus is the body and sexual positions. The typical fantasy woman in men's thoughts is lusty, sexually aroused easily and wants sex without strings attached.

Lesbian-love fantasies, or fantasies in which he and his partner bring another person into bed, are among the most common erotic voyages men take. It doesn't matter who the women are – just as long as he can sit back and have them ravish him and each other. This has nothing to do with your own sex capabilities or shortcomings. Researchers speculate that for many men, this fantasy may be a way to express the repressed feminine sides of their personalities. Subconsciously, they may be putting themselves into the role of one of the women – and thoroughly enjoying it.

At the same time, this fantasy gives him a break from his anxieties about having to take charge between the sheets. He can join in, or be passive and enjoy the show.

'She's gotta have it' is another common male fantasy theme. For a lot of men, dating and making love are fraught with rejection. These experiences leave a shadow of a doubt in many men's minds as to whether they're really desirable to women. So their subconscious has them conjuring up women who never, ever reject them.

Along the same lines is his fantasy of you having sex with other men. He'd be torn up if it happened in real life, but in fantasy, it says something about his worth. You're his woman. His. And if you're desirable, and you're his, that means he's got props. Having another man bring his girlfriend to orgasm also allows him to envision you sexually satisfied without putting the onus on himself to make it happen.

Adam, 27, software analyst

A threesome with two women – I guess that is every man's fantasy. I'd have a very HARD time watching two naked women lick each other's pussies without jumping in myself and joining them. I just imagine the beautiful sights and the wet sounds and I get hard as steel. I'd wish I had two cocks so I can fuck both of them at the same time! Oh, to feel my cock buried deep inside a wet, warm pussy and to have my tongue buried inside another ... wow!

I have had this thought almost nightly. Mainly wishful thinking as opposed to having it during masturbation or sex (which I don't have right now, unfortunately). Yes, I would like to have this fantasy come true! Can you arrange it?

Matthew, 30, air traffic controller

One of my best fantasies is my wife on top in a 69 with another woman while I fuck her from behind. The other girl's tongue would be on her pussy and my cock at the same time while she's going down on her.

Other things that get me: G-strings and thongs. Man, I'm an addict so seeing the women in those would be a total turn-on. I love it when you can see the lines of them through a woman's pants or skirt. I think I might like wearing them too.

Sam, 27, solicitor

Last night as I was stroking it, I fantasized being under a woman's total command. Though I have never had a bi experience, the thought of a woman ordering me to kiss another man's balls and cock really turns me on. First she ties us up and prick-teases us for what seems like hours, until she has us begging just to kiss her wet panties. She uses a dildo on herself in front of us, and then makes us lick her sweet juices off it, 'just for practice for the real thing later on,' she says. After having her way with us in everyway imaginable, she sits back and recovers. She then says for us to have a contest – the winner will receive a special 'treat'. She makes us write a short letter to her explaining why we want to suck on a cock and lick some balls. She then makes us give a demonstration on her dildo. The best letter and demonstration performed on her dildo will get to do the real thing. Of course, my letter and demonstration win, but she still commands me to do it, and though I seems real hesitant, she knows that I love every inch as it slides in my mouth.

Colin, 30, journalist

It is my dream to have sex in front of a paying audience of strangers. The idea of all those eyes ogling me and wanting me but not being able to touch me makes me rock hard. I hope that I might be able to make this fantasy a reality someday.

Anonymous

My fondest memories start at the age of 16. My elder brother, 22, recently married a Punjabi girl called Neetu. She was 19, roughly 36C-25-36, 5ft 5in, had long, knee length black hair plaited, white ivory coloured skin, a light shade of green bedroom eyes, tits that were so firm she hardly wore a bra, long shapely legs and firm but soft thighs and what an arse!

I had always fancied her even before the wedding, when her photo was sent to our family. She was wearing a tight traditional outfit enhancing her lovely curvaceous figure. Let's say I took the picture with me into the toilet more than a couple of times to jerk off.

She had a lovely personality too – very friendly and jokey. After the wedding, we would constantly tease each other and became good friends.

One day, I saw her changing. The door to my brother's room was slightly ajar and I saw her completely naked. I got an instant hard on. She bent over to towel her wet legs and I saw her pussy lips slowly being revealed from under her lovely, round arse the more she crouched. I could not help it. I started to masturbate as she gently towelled herself dry. I came against the blue doors when she turned around revealing her hairy bush and lovely slit. Luckily, she did not see me.

This became the basis of the fantasy I always have. I am walking down the hall and hear noises from my brother's old room. He is in there with his wife and she is being fucked raw by him. My eyes are completely focused on her body and reactions and noises of pleasure. This fucking slut has a side to her I have never seen. As you can imagine, I have dick in hand whilst watching the bitch of my dreams getting fucked senseless. Halfway through her fucking session it seems to me that she is looking in my direction making her actions aimed towards me. She is sucking my brother's dick with eager enthusiasm all the while looking in my direction, occasionally glancing in the mirror to see my cock's reaction. Eventually she is on her back, her tits jiggling like crazy. She is still looking in my direction as she brings her legs up to her chest, widening her cunt. She begins to moan a lot louder, still looking in my direction as she is being pounded. 'Oh yes! Fuck me! Make my pussy cum!' she moans. I come as the door closes.

Louis , 26, stock controller

This fantasy is based on something I once saw in a movie.

She is sitting at the bar, alone. I see her immediately when I walk in. I walk over to where she sits and stand close to her as I order a beer.

She touches my leg. 'I want you,' she says. 'I want you for the evening.'

Her fingers grow more insistent at that spot that makes my cock twitch. Smiling, she moves her hand over my cock, gently squeezing it through my jeans. I can't say a word as she strokes my cock under the bar, away from seeing eyes. She moves her hand, trailing it back down my inner thigh, back to hold her drink on the bar.

'There's just one thing. I call the rules. Whatever I say, whatever I need, you'll comply.'

I look at her. No one has ever propositioned me like this before.

'My name is Samantha. The rules are simple, really. You would be mine for the evening. Do whatever I want. Talk when I say you can, come when I allow you to.' She inhales her cigarette deeply, leans toward me, right breast grazing my upper arm. 'If you agree to be mine for the evening, you'll obey me.'

My excitement mounts. 'Alright. For the evening I will obey you.'

She stands up. 'Let's go.'

When we get to her car, she sits so I can see she's wearing no underwear. I stare, but she pushes my head back.

'Turn around and face the front. You'll not look at me again until I ask you to. Understood?'

'Yes,' I reply. 'I understand.'

We arrive at her house and I follow her in. She orders me to take a shower. My cock is standing straight out as I feel the water rushing over me.

'Don't move. I'll dry you off,' she says.

She picks up the towel and starting at the top of my shoulders, gently wipes the water from my back. As each area of my flesh is dried, she kisses it, slowly. By the time she gets to my ass, my body is shaking with anticipation. I don't expect the slap on my ass. Startled, I turn around, only to feel her hands on my hips, stopping me. 'Don't turn around.' She slaps my ass again, not enough to hurt me, yet enough to make me realize I have no choice.

She kisses the spots she slapped, gently nipping my ass with her teeth. I am having a hard time staying still. Her hands rub the towel over my chest and stomach, mouth following every inch of my body. Just as her next move is going to be on my cock, she stands up.

I feel her tongue on the base of my cock. I try to force myself deep into her mouth and feel the slight sting of her palm on my upper stomach. 'You can't come yet, you're not to move, you're not to speak,' she says.

She takes out a thick piece of silk from a dresser drawer and places it over my eyes. Her hands caress my nipples, rotating them in the palms of her hands. I feel a pinch, she's putting little clamps on my nipples. I'm not sure I like it and am about to say something when I feel her tugging at my balls while flicking the clamps. The feeling is intense. She takes me in her mouth. I am straining not to come. I feel my balls tighten. Finally, after what seems an eternity, she whispers, 'You can come now.' Her mouth covers my cock. Her tongue swirls my entire length as it slides deep into her throat.

Thomas, 29, sports management executive

I took an interest in this woman at work a few years ago. We talked openly and honestly about everything under the sun – sex included. One day she revealed to me that she had a rape fantasy. I couldn't believe it. She was smart, educated, and I thought all this talk about 'rape fantasies' was just a myth. So I asked her, 'You don't mean you want to be met by some thug in the parking lot wielding a knife and demanding to have sex with you, do you?'

She said 'No, of course not. I want to be thrown to the floor and "taken" by someone.'

That's when I did some research and came up with the word ravishment. Ravishment is what she wanted. She was tired of men making wimpy love to her; tired of hearing the question 'was that good for you?' Just once she'd like to know that a man wanted her so much at that moment that he couldn't help himself.

Our relationship was entirely chaste but I constantly fantasized about being the one to 'ravish' her.

In my favourite, we've walked around the city for hours before coming home. We don robes for comfort and I make her dinner. I steer the conversation to sex. I keep the conversation there until I can't stand the sexual tension. Then I tell her to go to the living room and I'll bring coffee.

And of course I don't bring coffee. I wait till she is half way there and run and grab her from behind, dropping her to the floor and ravishing her. No foreplay except for the sex talk. Just ramming into her. She is practically crying with joy. We explode at the same time.

Ian, 31, supervisor

Most frequently, I imagine a woman masturbating and getting really aroused. I don't know who she is, but she is very hot with big breasts and full hips and a wet pussy. In another, I am with my lover and she wakes up in the middle of the night and starts to seduce me. I imagine her getting out of control because she is so turned on.

Jim, 32, auctioneer

I have a lot of fantasies, but this is the one I masturbate most often to. The woman is based on someone I saw at work once. She wore a slinky black sheath dress with buttons down the front. In my fantasy, the last one-third are unfastened and I catch a glimpse of thigh every time she takes a step. Her legs are long and shapely and I can see she has stockings with garters fastened to the tops. I feel my manhood twitch in my pants. Her supple breasts bounce slightly as she moves towards me and I find myself unconsciously licking my lips as I watch them. My eyes wander down to her gently swaying hips.

I want her. No doubt about it. I don't care how or where, I just know I have to have her and now. I stand abruptly and meet her at the side of my desk in front of the soft leather couch. My fingers grip her forearms as she melts against my chest and I bow my head slightly to smell her hair. It smells of oranges. Oranges and cinnamon. She always smells good enough to eat, and that's exactly what I want to do. I lower her into the deep pillows of the couch and sink to my knees in front of her. She moans softly at my urgency and arches back.

I fumble with her buttons quickly, growing more and more anxious to devour her. Her sensual smell rises to my nose and I savour the aroma as inch by inch her luscious flesh is revealed to me. Her breasts are bare and I squeeze them gently on my way downward. I keep wondering when I will hit the top of her panties, but I never seem to. The garter belt is a satiny red material. My fingers caress it and a little smile spreads across my face as she whispers, 'I wore this just for you, Lover.'

My fingers continue the exotic journey until I feel a soft tuft of hair. Still no panty line. Then I suddenly realize she isn't wearing any and I almost tear the rest of the buttons from her dress to gain access to her heat. The last button releases and my two thick fingers slide down over her mound and disappear inside. She lets out a loud moan and spreads her legs wider for me to reach into her soft warmth more easily.

My tongue quickly finds her clit and I bathe it in my saliva, flicking quickly across the smooth red nub. Her excitement increases as I use all my expertise between her thighs. She writhes around on the soft seat and I take her legs one by one and slide them onto my shoulders. I pleasure her for a very long time. She becomes lost in a kind of euphoria. I know how to touch a woman in every way.

Her excitement rises and falls like a wild roller coaster ride and I tease her into submission. I move up her body finally and my mouth finds her eager nipples as my hard member slides into her delicious folds. I begin to pump against her hips and my mouth explores the rest of her body as my arm wraps around her thigh, still raised over my shoulder, and my fingertip rubs her hard clit.

She feels the heat between us and feels it spread through her pelvic rise. Her body begins to shudder and contract around me. It isn't long before I lose control and release inside her. She vibrates against my hipbones as multiple orgasms wash over her and I continue to tease the flesh between her legs. 'Don't stop', she whispers hoarsely, 'Don't ever stop. Mmmmmm!'

I smile at the obvious pleasure I am making her feel. I like having that power over her. I like that I can make her knees weak in a matter of seconds, or minutes or hours, whichever I choose. I know how to please her. How to make her nerve endings tingle with my touch. How to make her body respond to my gentle manipulations. She knows that I and only I can make her feel this way.

Larry

I am a medium-sized guy who has always loved the idea of watching his wife sucking a very large cock. I have two friends who occasionally visit us. One of the two has a very large circumcised member, the other has a small uncircumcised one (at least smaller than my average one). I am not circumcised myself. When they visit us, we often talk about sex and their wives don't seem to mind. Here is my fantasy. Unfortunately I have never acted upon it even though my wife would love the idea. The reason is I'm afraid of how my friends would react:

One day my two friends would come over without their wives. We would have a few drinks and as usual the talk would turn to sex. Suddenly my wife says, 'Let's play a game.' Without much fuss, she starts rubbing our crotches and asks us to stand up and stand next to each other. She unbuckles our belts and pulls down our pants.

Without comment, she gets a stack of newspapers and covers the floor in front of us. She commands us to masturbate while she watches and promises whoever shoots his load the farthest (as determined by cum spots on the newspaper) would get a blow job. We start masturbating feverishly; my wife watching with amusement. My well-endowed friend shoots first, his ejaculate shooting much further than our embarrassing driblets. As his reward, my wife goes down on him giving him a prolonged, noisy, very wet blow job, while we look on. With my friend's dick in her mouth she suddenly grabs our uncircumcised penises, pulls both of our foreskins back and starts rubbing our penis tips against each other. She then interrupts her blow job and pulls my friend's foreskin over the head of my penis. I become very hard and turn bright red in my face because I have got a hard-on from being in contact with another man's dick in front of my wife.

My wife then tells all three of us to stand close to each other. With both hands she grabs our three penises, shoves all three of them into her mouth and starts sucking and slurping until we all come. She then tells us to clean up the mess and leave.

That's my fantasy. I wonder whether it is shared by many husbands.

Arnold, 33, insurance under-writer

This is the fantasy I think about when I'm masturbating. An ex-girlfriend of mine is standing in a bar when she suddenly grabs hold of the bartender. All other activity on the bar stops as they push against each other against the bar and start shagging madly on top of it. Everyone starts pulling her clothes off of her and pawing at her. She moans loudly with pleasure.

Jim, 25, sales executive

I'm tied to a four-poster bed while two women in sexy lingerie are having sex at the end of the bed. I lie there waiting for them to finish, but my turn doesn't come for hours. Eventually they pour oil all over my body and rub their bodies against my slippery skin until I come. This is one of my favourite fantasies. I even had to play with myself while writing it!

Mark, 28, waiter

I'm driving in an open-top car, up above the sky is blue and there's just me and this girl who's definitely Posh Spice. The roads are all empty and as she drives and changes gears, her skirt starts to ride up her thighs. Every now and then we get too fired up to continue driving and pull over to have sex on the bonnet, the back seat, even against the door. Then we start driving again, with music blaring out of the stereo.

Graham 25, graphic designer

I'm having sex with a woman who has breasts so big I can't hold them in two hands. She grabs my head and plunges my face between them. I am surrounded by their softness. Then she demands that I lick them and bite her nipples until she tells me to stop. They feel so huge in my hands and I love playing with them. She then positions me so my penis is between her breasts and enveloped by them. We have sex this way. When it's over, I fall asleep with my head on her breasts.

Neil, 26, photographer

I suppose it's a macho thing but I fantasize about satisfying two women at once. My fantasy goes like this: I'm in a pub and two girls, who are friends, both try to chat me up. They're not planning a ménage à trois, they think I'll pick the one I fancy. But I like them both and ask them both back for a night-cap. I take one of them into the shower with me and when the other comes looking for us, she strips off and says she doesn't want to miss the action. Basically, I'm being lathered up and taken advantage of by these two gorgeous girls. While I'm bonking one girl, the other is touching her and I watch them pleasing each other.

Tim, 22, student

I have the same fantasy with some variations. While I'm asleep, this woman, a stranger, lets herself into my house and comes into my bedroom. I don't hear her but wake up to her giving me a blow job. As I look down at her body, she's wearing a leather mini skirt and thigh-length patent black boots. She handcuffs me and ties me to the bed. Next thing, she's on top of me demanding that I satisfy her. It's bloody amazing. Every time I'm about to come she stops what she is doing and moves on to something else. Then she sits on my face and I imagine smelling her leather skirt while having oral sex. I don't do any of these things in any particular order and usually run out of time to think about them all before I come. But basically I like the thought of being dominated by a woman I don't know.

Tony, 26, marketing assistant

When I was 16, I fancied my mate's mum. I still fantasize about being taken in hand by an older woman, though it's not her nowadays. It's not anybody, really, just someone who is sexually experienced, confident and demanding. She does things like whip a vibrator out of a drawer and shows me how to use it on her. It's like she's giving me the most erotic biology lesson of my life. She's not shy in any way and is really explicit. She tells me exactly what women like done to them and then I do it.

I did once have a fling with a married woman so I think about that sometimes, though I have to embellish it and make her older.

Simon, 26, accountant

I get arrested by a female police officer who takes me into an interview room and seduces me. She starts saying that I need to be taught a lesson. She gets out her handcuffs and undresses me, before getting on top. I'm naked but she leaves her uniform on, including her knickers, which is a real turn-on. This adds a sense of urgency and furtiveness, which gives me a major erection.

The turn-on here is that she knows she should be professional but because I'm so damned irresistible, she throws all her professionalism out the window. I like the power I have over her to turn her into a sex fiend. Obviously this is a fantasy I'd never live out and probably wouldn't want to.

Craig, 27, laboratory technician

I'd never have the courage to go to a prostitute but it doesn't stop me fantasizing about it. I would just pull up to a curb and she gets in. She's wearing boots, a plastic shiny mac and nothing on underneath. We drive off to a secluded street and then she asks what services I require. 'The best blow job in the world,' I say and that's what I get. I like the fact that it's really business-like and there's no emotional attachment. I can tell her exactly how I want it without feeling embarrassed or critical.

It doesn't mean that I don't want to be emotionally attached to women I have relationships with in real life. I just want a quick no questions fuck sometimes.

Ethan, 25, insurance broker

Once a female client came into the office for a meeting wearing a shortish skirt and no knickers. I couldn't believe it, she was sitting opposite me and subtly crossing and uncrossing her legs. I could see everything. It was exciting and scary at the same time. I kept thinking what I would do I'd do if my colleagues weren't there. I turned it into a fantasy when I got home. After the meeting she asks to have a word in private and, with a raging hard-on, I lock the door and give her one on the boardroom table.

Carl, 25, data programmer

I meet this girl in a pub and she comes home with me. We open a bottle of wine, start groping each other and end up rubbing against each other on the carpet. She undresses and hands me her underwear. I start to put it on the floor, but she says, 'No, YOU put it on.' It's a silk shirt and black lacy knickers. I'm shocked at first but I give in when she makes it clear nothing else will go on until I do.

She starts rubbing the silk over my body with her hands and the feel of it really turns me on. Then she fondles me through these tight little knickers while easing her fingers up the sides and inside them. She's getting really turned on and keeps telling me how horny it is. Then she bends down and starts removing the knickers with her teeth. When they're off, she takes the shirt off me and starts giving me a hand job using the silk. It's so amazing I come in five seconds flat.

Grant, 24, credit controller

I have holiday fantasies. In one, I'm skiing with my mates. They're all on the slopes but I've got a bad hangover and can't get up in time, I'm lying on top of the bed stark naked when the chalet maid bursts in the door. She's about 18, blond, Swedish and cute. She asks if it's okay to clean the room, not even seeming to notice I have no clothes on. I say yes. She starts tidying up around me and I start masturbating watching her. She goes into the bathroom and cleans it, but walks out with no clothes on. She says that she'd like to finish the job for me, grips me gently in her hand and bends down to kiss and lick my balls.

The other holiday story is on a plane. I'm flying first class on my own. The air hostess keeps bending over me with a low-cut dress on, asking me if I'd like anything. Finally, she comes over and says I look a bit pale and would I like to lie down for a while in her private cabin. She locks me in with her and shags me senseless.

Dominic, 32, executive

I have to travel a lot for work. I often get horny and watch one of those porno movies on the hotel telly. Afterwards, I imagine someone lying down on top of me. I don't care what the sex is, I am so hard. If it's a man, I'd feel his cock sink between my buttocks as he lowered his weight. With a woman, the soft tickle of her pubic hair on my ass just before her loins and hips enveloped me.

Steve, 32, investment banker

My co-worker is the sexiest thing I have ever seen. I have spent many hours in my office with this fantasy when I should have been working!

She walks into the room. Her long auburn hair falls about her shoulders in soft tendrils, rubbing up and down her bare shoulders, and teasing across her ample cleavage as she moves. She smiles as I look up at her and I lay down my pen and sit back in my desk chair. She walks slowly, sensually across the room and with each step I can feel my temperature rise.

I wonder what will happen if my secretary accidentally walks in on us. I think perhaps she knows better than to interrupt me when she is there though. It is obvious, the way we feel about each other.

I sit looking at her. She undoes her dress until her nearly naked body is exposed. She sits on the couch in my office, raises her feet to the edge and spreads her legs giving me a clear view of her moist slit below the red garter belt. The lacy tops of her silky stockings frame her delicate folds. I sigh a great heaving sigh and touch myself lightly. My member begins to rise slowly, twitching as the blood rushes to the head and the pressure makes me ooze slightly.

She lowers her right hand and cups her sex. She massages slowly, sensually as I watch intently. She undulates her fingers against her opening until she begins to feel the excitement again between her thighs. It feels so good. She continues as I watch and soon slides a finger into herself and then another. That feels even better and she soon takes up a rhythm. I fight the urge to go to her and gently tug on my hard cock. It grows rigid with my effort and I soon find myself moaning.

She stands and walks over to me, lowering herself between my legs, in front of my chair. I lean back and open my legs wide in anticipation. I love to feel her mouth envelope me. Love to watch her bright red lipstick swallow me up and try to pull me in deeper. Her tongue is strong and seems to find the inner secrets I try to hide. My head is swollen and quivers at her touch. I want to flood her mouth with my cream and watch as she swallows every drop. She knows how to drive me to the brink of madness and pull me safely back.

She plays me like a fine instrument. I am completely under her spell. I think I can hear music in my head, beating to the rhythm of her movements and echoed only by my own animal-istic sounds. I growl and groan and moan under my breath as her mouth works me into a frenzy. My hips pump upward, gently but firmly, trying to drive my shaft deeper into the back of her throat. She seems to swallow me up and my body quiv-ers each time I watch myself disappear into those delectable lips of hers.

Her hands are not idle. They move about my landscape, exploring all the tenderest parts, urging me ever onward into an ecstasy I never knew existed. I feel my nerve endings tingle, from my toes all the way up to my scalp and to my outer extremities. I feel I will either go crazy or implode if I don't release soon. She brings me to the brink and then squeezes me at my base to make me retreat from the brink of orgasm.

She does this over and over until she thinks I have had enough and then she allows my release. I lie back against the firm chair back and wait for that incredible warmth to flow through my loins and surge up my shaft to splash across her thirsty tongue. She drinks me in quickly and moans at my taste.

When my body relaxes finally she lays her head in my lap and I begin petting her long auburn hair back out of her face. My fingers feel good against her velvety cheeks and I stroke across her temple and down her neck. My fingertips stop now and then to caress her earlobe. She is enjoying the attention and doesn't make any attempt to move.

The phone rings a moment later and I begin chatting with a co-worker in another part of the building. I say I am taking a little coffee break and will he meet me later to discuss the details of a project he is working on. I chuckle softly at the reply I receive and smile down at her, with her head still nestled in my lap.

Phil, 29, investment banker

I'm hiding in the closet, watching this woman get ready for bed. She has red hair and is tall and muscular, very unlike the sort of women I usually go for. She's putting on sexy lingerie, even though she's alone. I spring out, overpower her and start having sex with her.

At first, she fights. But mid-way through, she becomes overwhelmed by my sexual skills and becomes incredibly aroused and surrenders to me. We both continue to a powerful orgasm.

Grub

My favourite fantasy involves having a threesome with my wife and another man. My best friend is really well hung (we go to the same gym) and I would love to watch her squirm under him while he pounds away. After he blows his load into her, I would dive between her legs and lick her pussy clean of his come.

I would also like to suck his big cock and fuck his ass while she watches.

I think this is an attainable fantasy because the three of us were drunk at a Christmas party and while she was under the mistletoe he grabbed her and kissed her passionately while I watched. He also copped a feel. My wife has big tits and was wearing a low cut gown. Fortunately, no one else was around.

Just thinking of that scene makes me unbelievably horny. My wife gets embarrassed when I bring it up and my friend says he can't remember, or so he claims.

Ben, 32, engineer

I awake and I am in bed with a woman who is not my wife. I don't know how I have ended up there – whether I got too drunk and picked her up or if she is a prostitute.

The woman gives a long murmur of pure pleasure. Her arm reaches out, grasping my shaft hotly. She gives a soft, sleepy chuckle.

'Mmm, ready for me again?' Her voice drips with sensuality. She slides a long thigh over me and lifts herself easily astride my hips. The sheet falls away and I drink in the glory of her nakedness. She is tanned and lithe, breasts full and firm, nipples dark and puckered. Her face is sultry and oozing with lust, her lips swollen and moist.

She slides her hot juiced slit up and down the length of my cock, rubbing her clit hard along me. She is shaved and smooth, quite unlike my wife.

'You amaze me,' she croons. 'How many times was it last night? Eight, I counted. And three in my ass.' As she speaks, she sits back to impale herself on my column. I moan loudly at the feel of her hot tightness sliding down my cock.

'Oh God, you're so big!' she purrs. 'Yes! Fill me up!'

I watch cross-eyed as my mighty cock disappears into her sleek body. She surrounds me with her hot, wet cavern, her muscles tugging me in deeper. She begins to ride me, bouncing up and down faster and faster, my cock-head hitting hard against her cervix on every stroke.

This is raw sex like I have never experienced it. The woman leans back, holding my knees with her hands, rasping my cock against the front of her vagina, and howls with delight as I stretch her wide. She begins to shudder and writhe, mewling in the throes of approaching orgasm. For me, accustomed to a wife who had silent climaxes, if at all, it's too thrilling to stand. I explode inside her with a violence that shocks me.

I must fill every crevice of her insides with my first few jets, for soon foamy white semen began to spurt out around the shaft of my cock, soaking my pubic hair and covering her mons and thighs. I feel the convulsive contractions of her cunt milking all my seed from my balls.

Eventually we are spent and she just sits there, her sweat-covered breasts rising and falling, still holding me in her.

Daniel, 32, security officer

In my fantasy I am in bed and naked – I usually sleep in pyjamas. I have an erection, but it is different, harder, potent – as if it had been solid all night. When I reach down to touch it, I realize it is easily twice the length and girth of my usual rather average specimen. It is a solid hot cylinder of raw power, ridged and veined, pulsing with life, irresistibly strokeable. My heart rate increases with a mixture of fear and excitement.

I manage to take my hands off my cock, with which I have already fallen in love, to explore other bits of my body. I am more muscular, a hairier chest, no soft belly caused by too much food and not enough exercise. I feel fitter, energetic.

I return to my cock, unable to keep my hands off of it. I spend the rest of the day stroking myself to orgasm after orgasm. It is inexhaustible.

Billy, 26, entertainment planner

I am so big I can give myself a blow job. I imagine fingering my cock. A clear drop squeezes from the slit. I catch it with my right forefinger and dab it on my tongue. I bend over and take myself in my mouth.

With my thumb and middle finger, I give my nipples short, quick tweaks, like snapping my fingers.

I roll over onto my stomach. I pull down so the foreskin reveals the head. Up and down a few times, squeezing hard. I pump my cock hard and I feel close to coming and angle my cock up so that I'll empty into my mouth. I raise my hips off the rug, arch my back, and come. A couple of strong spasms yield quickly to weak twitches. The semen jets out twice, three times. I swallow and go to sleep.

David, 29, legal advisor

Every time I drive by that old Victorian home on Elmwood Avenue I have the same hot thought. The house where one grows up is usually packed with endless memories, but in my case only one came to mind. It has to do with my little sister Kerry.

Kerry's nickname was 'Princess' because she was so pretty. Even after we were in college, I sometimes used her nickname.

Kerry and I were only 10 months apart in age (I was the oldest) and were unusually close for a brother and sister. We had our share of squabbles all right, but that's only normal. What wasn't quite normal, however, were the feelings I started getting for Kerry in college. Looking back, I can't exactly pinpoint the moment when I stopped seeing Kerry as a sister and saw her as an extremely sensuous, very desirable young woman. When we'd get together during our visits home from different colleges, I'd find myself staring at her ass or licking my lips over her tits. I started fantasizing about her when I masturbated, and there were even a couple of occasions when I started getting aroused just from being in the same room with my sister!

It was all very confusing. But at the same time it was exciting and exhilarating. The orgasms I had after jacking off with images of Kerry in my head were the best I ever had. I should mention that modesty was never a big priority in our family. We didn't exactly walk around naked in front of each other but no one thought anything about being seen in their underwear. Since I'd started having these feelings for Kerry, I'd been hoping for a glimpse of my sister in bra and panties, but it never happened.

This is my favourite Kerry fantasy.

Kerry has been out on a date and comes in a bit tipsy on Margaritas. We always chat after dates if the other one's light is still on. My light isn't on when Kerry reels home this night, but she comes in anyway. I am fast asleep and the next thing I know someone tumbles into bed beside me and starts tickling me.

'Kerry! What the hell? You're drunk!' 'Not drunk, David,' she says. 'Just pleasantly horny.' She is more than horny, and her good mood is contagious. She starts tickling me again, and before I know it I have kicked half the covers off. I always sleep in the raw, and in the craziness of Kerry's tickling, my dick gets exposed a couple of times. She points it out of course, with much laughter, and then it becomes a game for her to really get a look. I might indulge her under other circumstances, but with her crawling all over me I start getting aroused. The more she rubs her body against mine, pressing her big boobs against my bare chest and kissing me playfully, my dick is getting harder by the moment. There is no way I am going to let her see me with an erection. Or am I? My head is spinning with the possibilities. After all, I think, she is the one who is instigating all this craziness.

Still, I think, she's not in complete control and might not remember everything. But as these thoughts go through my mind, I don't have a chance to act on them because Kerry makes a sudden powerful lunge and pulls the sheets down to my knees. My big dick bursts into view, all eight inches fully erect and pointed right at the ceiling. I start to shove the pillow over my lap until I see the look on Kerry's face. 'Damn, David!' she gasps, a hand going automatically to her breast. 'That's the most beautiful cock I've ever seen!' 'Is it?' I ask, with amazing calm. 'Yes,' she says, leaning over for a closer look. It was as if she is inspecting a piece of art, and I am almost amused at the way she looks at it with a critical eye. 'It's a lot thicker than Steven's. Longer too.' (I think, well, that solves the mystery about whether she's sleeping with her boyfriend or not.) 'And look at those big balls!' 'C'mon, Ker,' I say, finally getting embarrassed. 'You make me feel like a prize bull at a county fair.'

'Well, maybe that's how I see you just now,' she replies. She frowns for a minute as she stares at my dick and then she remembers she is still wearing her heavy coat. She takes it off and gives me a quizzical look. 'Turn about's fair play, don't you think, David?' 'Uh, sure.' I don't know what she means, but I watch breathlessly as she unbuttons her blouse and tosses it aside. Her bra goes next, and I gasp again as she loosens those beautiful tits of hers and lets them swing free. She must've worn a really confining bra because her tits are much bigger than I'd thought. I'm not exaggerating when I say she could've been a centrefold, her young body is that perfect! 'What do you think?' she asks, cupping her big boobs together and lifting them to her face.

My dick twitches when I see my sister lick her own nipples and flick her tongue in my direction. 'Wow!' It is all I can manage. There is more to come. While Kerry ogles my crotch, she slithers out of her skirt and takes a few minutes to let me enjoy seeing her in just her panties. Again I think she is real centrefold material, especially when she strikes a few provocative poses for my benefit. When she rubs her crotch with both hands and licks her lips, I just about lose control. 'Ready for the unveiling?' she teases. She hooks her thumbs in her panties and pulls them down a couple of inches. 'Oh, yeah!' I say. Kerry gets to her feet and leans against the headboard, her crotch just inches from my face.

I can smell her pussy, and the sweet scent almost makes me dizzy. I love the aroma of cunt and can't resist leaning closer so that I can rub my nose in the nylon of my sister's panties. I feel Kerry grab my head and hold on as she shoves forward with her hips. My tongue licks against that thin nylon barricade between her juicy pussy and my cunt-hungry mouth. 'Yes,' she sighs. 'Yes!' Soon I have Kerry's panties dripping wet with my spit and can see the dark bush beneath the pink nylon.

I can't stand the teasing any more and reach for the waistband of her panties. Slowly I pull them down, baring the 'V' of brunette pubic hairs pointing toward my goal. Finally those panties are down around my sister's knees and she wriggles carefully out of them. 'What a beautiful cunt!' I cry. 'And it's all for you, David,' she whispers. I grab Kerry by the ass and pull her closer. She opens her legs to welcome my tongue, and finally I am tasting what I've been after all along. It is delicious. She comes again and again.

SEX FANTASIES BY WOMEN FOR WOMEN

sharing
your fantasies

Introduction

The feedback on sharing your sexual fantasies is mixed. The experts advise you to tread carefully, saying that generally your sexual fantasies are best kept private – a secret part of your life where your deepest wishes, hopes, fears, angers and other emotions are expressed. It seems that not only can sharing be loaded with embarrassment, studies have discovered that many people find when they share their spiciest fantasy, the whole thing fizzles instead of sizzles.

That said, those same experts have found that revealing sexual fantasies can be fun, sexy, spice up the relationship, add excitement and draw partners closer together. But they stress that occurs only if there's a high level of intimacy, commitment and trust between the couple.

If you do decide to have a true confessions fantasy moment with your lover, one word of advice: slowly work your way up the erotica ladder. No matter how long you've been together, you may find yourself feeling embarrassed or threatened if he suddenly expresses interest in the woman with big breasts on

Page 3 while he wonders if his penis measures up after hearing about how you long to be caressed by a bevy of women. And stress that it's just a fantasy and there's no need to act it out, unless you both want to and feel comfortable doing that.

Suzanna, 31, graphic designer

My boyfriend has this fantasy where I am a virgin he seduces. It took him a long time to tell me about it, but now we talk about it every time we make love. It turns us both on and has lots of variations – sometimes, he is a sultan and I am his slave. In another, I am a little girl and he is my teacher. My favourite is when we pretend to be teenagers playing doctor.

Michele, 26, engineer

Sometimes my boyfriend and I make up this fantasy where he is someone else. It can be someone we know or a celebrity. Our best is when he pretends he is my boss and I get to order him around. We thought about making it real once – I would seduce my boss while my boyfriend hid and watched – I know my boss has the hots for me so it wouldn't have been hard. But the reality did not seem like it could be as sexy as what we had made up. I'm glad we decided not to do it as I don't think I could have looked my boss in the eye afterwards.

Danielle, 32, DJ

I have lots of fantasies – being pinned down against my will, making love standing up, ravishing some man I think is gorgeous.

Recently, I've started sharing my fantasies with my partner and we both find it very exciting. I think about taking him, being the one who seduces him and does everything, just using him as a sort of living dildo until he gets so excited that he has to move. He talks about me screwing him to the point where he is left gasping for breath. He also likes my fantasy about being with lots of men and him watching.

I don't think we would ever act them out though, because I don't think it would be as hot in reality.

Belinda, 21, student

When I revealed to my boyfriend a fantasy of a simultaneous coupling with two foreign exchange students in my class, he said, 'Go for it, but if you do, don't come back.' He meant it. He didn't want to hear what I was fantasizing about and found the whole thing sordid. Since then, he hasn't really trusted me and asks me where I go when I am out on my own and who I am with.

Paula, 31, medical equipment sales

My favourite fantasy is being intimate with two sexy male prostitutes at the same time. When I shared it with my husband, he called me a 'sick pervert'. Ever since, I think he doesn't really trust me. And now the fantasy doesn't work for me any more either.

Isobel, 24, entertainment planner

My favourite fantasy dates back to when I was around 13 and first discovered the magic of masturbation. It was all about being a kidnapped maiden, tied up in this elaborate but revealingly ripped gown. Just as the villain is about to attack me, the hero comes in and whisks me off to some quiet secluded spot where we make love. The fantasy grew more elaborate as I became more experienced and I sometimes fall back on it during sex when I can't seem to get in the mood. But ever since I told my lover about it, the romance has sort of fallen flat. I have a new fantasy about being an 18th century virgin now which I intend to keep to myself!

Joan, 27, mother

I really mourned in my marriage that I was never going to have the wild sex I had before marriage. When I got married, I told my husband, 'I don't believe in passion dying – if it dies I'm going to be out of here.' But then it happened anyway, and of course I didn't leave. Then this year I went to see an old friend who revealed she was in a relationship with a woman, and having all this great sex. Driving home, I began having wild fantasies about my husband, like those I had when we were first together. When I got back, I told him what my friend had said and how it made me feel. We had the best sex I've ever had in my entire life. The funny thing was that for me, the fantasy that inspired such great sex was about my husband, and for him, it was about my girlfriend and her female lover.

Fiona, 24, painter

My boyfriend is hot to have a threesome with some women we know, and it gets me excited but recently I told him I wanted to have a threesome with another guy or a foursome. I would love to see him try sucking a cock and would also like him to get fucked in the ass while he and I '69' each other. He's not into it and doesn't even want to make up a fantasy about it. I think he thinks I am sick to want to pretend such a thing.

Jan, 29, retail manager

My fiancé and I regularly make up fantasies together. It makes our sex life more exciting, This is one of our favourites. I hope we can make it come true one day.

We usually sleep naked together because we find it comfortable. My fiancé frequently rubs my body because it helps me fall asleep. In our fantasy, he massages my vagina and upper thighs enough to arouse me while I am sleeping. Then he slowly begins to have sex with me so that I don't really wake up and instead remain in a dreamy, wonderful state. He wants me to have a wet dream, but initiated by him. I don't know why this is a fantasy of mine, but it is. I told him and he said that he'd try but that I would most likely wake up or roll over or something.

Gabrielle, 25, stylist

I have this fantasy whenever I get a massage. Recently I shared it with my lover and we have acted it out with him playing the part of my masseuse. It isn't quite the same, but it still makes me come every time – which straightforward, no-fantasy sex doesn't.

The fantasy starts as I get undressed and get on the table, draping a sheet over my lower back that falls just to mid-thigh. The door opens and a very attractive man walks in. He pours some oil into his hands and starts rubbing gently. I close my eyes, and try letting my mind focus on the sensations as his hands slide over my shoulders, down to the small of my back, just brushing lightly over the rise of my buttocks.

He starts working his way up my legs in a slow, sensual rhythm. I have now completely surrendered to the sensations coursing through my body.

As his hands slide over my thighs I moan slightly out loud, not able to keep it in. I press my groin hard against the table, feeling my wetness press against it. His hands slide further up my legs, slipping between them, inching closer to the place I desperately want him to touch.

He asks if I'm enjoying myself, and it's all I can do not to gasp my reply. He tells me he occasionally gives full-body massages, wondering if I'm interested. I agree immediately. He pulls the sheet from my body and, using the oil, he massages my ass, his fingers slipping between my legs, just brushing my pussy. I sigh and press back against his fingers as they slide away, once more brushing my legs lightly.

Gently, he turns me over, exposing my body to him. He pours more oil between my breasts, fingers spreading it in circles around them. The circles close in as his fingers approach my nipples. Then, teasingly, he starts at my feet, slowly working his way up. As his hands slide higher up my legs, I press hard against his fingers, feeling them push slowly into me. Two fingers slide inside, his thumb pressing against my clit. I arch against him, my orgasm taking control of my body.

He steps away from me, watching me writhe on the table in ecstasy. Then, murmuring for me to call him the next time I'm feeling stressed, he leaves the room, leaving me to gather my wits.

Nan, 25, masseuse

Sometimes during sex, I mentally morph my husband into Sylvester Stallone, Arnold Schwarzenegger, Jean Claude Van Damme – or a hunka-hunka fusion of all three. His arms and chest swell into strapping, heave-ho pistons of testosterone-pumping power. I, in turn, feel tiny, temptingly gorgeous, a seductress. I've told my husband about these fantasies and sometimes he encourages me to call him by the name of whomever I am fantasising about. It makes our lovemaking really sexy.

Another fantasy I have that I haven't told him about is being lovingly seduced by all of the Spice Girls. I just don't think he'd be able to handle me being with another woman – it would freak him out and make him think I am a lesbian, which I am definitely not. I'd never want to be with a woman in real life. But the idea of it is very sexy to me because I think a woman would know EXACTLY how to turn me on without any prompts from me.

Victoria, 28, nurse

I imagine I am living in a nineteenth century romance novel, where no one needs to go to work or is worried about deadlines or faxes, etc. My lover and I spend time making love and touching and kissing and talking. He joins me in the kitchen while I cook wonderfully sensual feasts. We feed each other, taking our time, licking one another's fingers and hands and lips, and then we begin making love before we've even finished our food. We sit in front of the fire drinking tea and giving each other foot massages. Occasionally, we take a walk by the lake, drinking in its splendid beauty and some wonderful fall sunsets, always ending in us making love.

I recently shared this fantasy with my lover. Since then, he has elaborated on it and turned himself into a sexy knight who saves me from danger, after which I give myself to him in gratitude. I am lucky to be with a guy who is so in tune with me. We even put on period fancy dress to keep the fantasy going.

Angela, 30, writer

My boyfriend and I live 300 miles from each other. This means that a lot of our relationship is over the phone or e-mail. Suffice to say, phone and 'web' sex keep us going. This is a letter I wrote to my lover about an imagined moment between us. We read it to each other over the phone regularly and masturbate as we do.

I knead your overworked muscles with my expert fingers. I touch even the deepest chords and soothe the ache within. My hands work quickly and dart off on some playful detour here and there as I work my way up and down your body. My hands are warm and delicious against your flesh.

Touching your body quickly arouses you and each of my senses is coaxed into readiness. I smell your musky scent beneath my fingers. I hear your low moans with each caressing movement. I see your arousal and marvel at the pink, erect reminder of your manhood. I feel my nerve endings react to the sights, sounds, smells and touch of you. I can't seem to get enough, and I surround your more than willing penis with my red painted nails and begin gently stroking up and down its length, daring it to grow thicker and more rigid.

Tiny beads form on the smooth head and I sample it with the tip of my tongue. Your body quivers at the sight and touch, and I smile at you and give you a sexy wink. I continue to play with your glistening shaft, licking it gently each time it dribbles, until I think you might be close to orgasm, then I back off and kiss your chest or your thighs until I feel you are under control again.

After teasing you for a long time I straddle your pelvis and slowly lower myself onto your shaft as you watch. You moan with pleasure at the sight and feel as my body squeezes around your thick shaft and it disappears inside. You lift your knees to drive yourself deeper and thrust upward each time I rock on you. It turns you on even more to watch my body swaying and rocking above you and to watch the pleasure on my face.

I'm lost in the motion. I ride you fiercely as your hands grope to find a firm hold and find none. Everything is motion. Fluid and ever changing. We become lost in it until the final wave explodes our sea of passion into a million tiny puddles and we lay spent again for the moment.

We lie side by side, spoons style, breathing in a sort of jagged rhythm, trying to pace each other back to something in a normal range. I feel the dewy sweat of our repeated copulation clinging to your body and brushing against mine. My senses are heightened now. Like a heat seeking missile, I feel you rise to the occasion yet again and smile secretly to myself.

My body hungers to feel you inside me, yet again. I can't get enough. As if in an alcoholic stupor, I seek out that one more drink, but it isn't a drink I lust after. It's your long, slick manliness. You sense my urgent lust and draw me quickly to my knees, my face close to the tile. My knees are together making a tight entrance for your slick member. You linger at my thighs, rubbing yourself gently against me, arousing my already active nerve endings, and then slowly slip between my soft lips.

I moan gently as you enter, swaying my hips back and forth to the music in the background. Slow and sensual and deep is how I want it and you seem to read my thoughts, being extra careful to follow my body movements and the music. When the music reaches a peak you thrust deeper into me with each crescendo. I rock back on you from time to time to meet your thrusts. The music begins to build and we both step up our motion until we again get lost in the passion and we both explode in orgasmic ecstasy and then collapse on the floor again. Your body covers mine, skin against skin, warm where it touches and cool where it doesn't. It's hard to believe we've made love to each other so many times and in so many ways and never got near a bed.

I let you catch your breath and then shimmy out from under you. I stand and take your hand, raising you up by sheer will, because I'm certainly not strong enough to lift you. You back me against the counter and your mouth comes down on mine with great force. Your passion is almost overwhelming. It takes my breath away for a moment and I find I'm light-headed. When you finally release me, I bury my nose in your chest and take in great deep breaths of you and of whatever oxygen might be clinging to the air around you. The dizziness subsides and I pull you towards the bathroom.

I reach into the tub and turn on the water faucets one by one, then turn to open a drawer and pull out a box of matches, striking one on the side of the box and touching it to the wicks of several candles. I close the door and turn to you, reaching behind my head to dowse the light and let the flickering candle-light engulf us.

Your face softens immediately and I think what a handsome creature you really are, among all that tousled hair. I see the love in your eyes and remember who and where I am with great clarity. We forgot for a little time, but now reality reminds us as we sink slowly into the warm water of the tub.

Chrissy, 29, computer sales

If I see a sexy man, I usually fantasize about what he looks like under those clothes. Are his thighs thick and firm? What's his penis like? I imagine him coming up and seducing me – and feeling his body against me with a bulge at the crotch. I also wonder what his skin and hair feel like and what he smells and tastes like.

My boyfriend and I are very open about these things and talk about different people we find sexy regularly, imagining together what sex would be like with them. It adds excitement to our love life, which might otherwise be stale after five years!

Rowena, 31, receptionist

This fantasy is based on something that actually happened with my boyfriend. He and I regularly re-live the episode, embellishing it or just remembering bits of it when we make love.

The sun was setting as I got into his car. It was a convertible and the top was down. As I got in, he asked me to remove my panties from underneath my short cotton sundress.

I slid into the black leather seat, adjusting the seatbelt. I glanced over at him and smiled. He was so handsome with his thick black hair and his tanned skin. His long, sleek body stretched behind the wheel. He popped the car into second and then third. 'We're going for a ride in the country babe,' he said quietly, 'I want you to lean back and relax.'

The car hugged the road as the sun went down behind the trees. The sky was orange and pink and the wind blew gently at my neck. I could smell the summer flowers as we drove quickly out of town. The air was laden with warmth as the summer day finished its journey. I felt myself escaping into the freedom of the road.

I closed my eyes, taking in his scent and feeling my growing desire in my groin. I longed to touch myself but felt too lazy. As if reading my mind, he reached over and gently put his hand on my thigh. The warmth and strength of his hand, mingling with the cool night air, made my body shiver with anticipation. He crept his hand up even higher, to my shaved box. I started to moisten with anticipation.

I desperately wanted him to touch me, yet he didn't. My hands reached to my breasts as I began to rub them quietly. And then I found myself inside the dress, twirling and pinching my nipples one at a time until the intensity and need of my desire was overwhelming.

I slid down deeper into the seat, and felt one, then two fingers inside me. He was barely looking at the road as he took my hardened clit into his hand and rubbed it gently. The more he rubbed, the wetter I got and when I couldn't stand the shuddering, I glanced at him. He was smiling, yet concentrating on what he was doing to me that was driving me wild. He continued to rub me, massaging my clit, feeling my cum, and the taking the wetness to rub my clit once more. I arched my back and pushed myself deeper into his hands.

'Yeah, baby, that's the way I like it,' he growled, 'make my hands wet with your desire, don't hold back, cum for me.'

As if the command was all I needed, my body exploded and my orgasm made a scream catch in my throat. I felt myself squirting and cuming over and over again.

At first I didn't hear him stop the car or turn off the ignition. I was aware of the darkness and the stars but my sexual high was blanketing me. He reached over and pressed the button that allowed my seat to recline. Climbing over me gracefully, he lifted my dress and placed his head down between my legs. Licking my hardness, I felt myself tightening again, wanting to fill his mouth with cum, wanting to touch him as well, yet not ever wanting him to stop. He licked me from the back to the front, pausing at my asshole as he encircled it with his tongue.

Hiking my dress up further he exposed my naked pussy to the air. The coolness of the air shocked my body at first but the warmth of his tongue brought me back. He braced himself so that his body was above me and I could feel his cock against my thighs through his pants. I reached out to touch his hardness. It felt so good.

Sliding under him I switched positions so that he was the one on the reclining seat. Gently I pushed his body back so that I could release him. Pulling at the zipper in one swift move, I grabbed his cock. It was hard and hot and I loved the way he looked. I bent down and flicked my tongue on the head. Encircling the head with the whole of my tongue, I pressed my fingernails into the shaft. I ran his cock across my lips and then placed the wholeness in my mouth. Spurts of cum came off the top and I licked them gingerly, holding his balls with my other hand as I did so. I took his cock and rubbed it against the roof of my mouth, and then down my throat once more. My lips wrapped around him and I listened as he moaned quietly.

I reached under his shirt and grabbed one nipple. Pinching it, while I sucked, I felt him twist and turn. He grabbed my hair and pulled at it as I took his entire cock down my throat. Licking and sucking, I felt him growing harder. I wanted him to explode but I wanted to ride him. I released him from my mouth and ran my tongue up his belly, toward his nipples while I kissed each one, sucking them until they were so erect I thought he was going to burn.

'Fuck me,' he whispered and shivers ran down my spine.

I hoisted my dress over my head and positioned my body so that I could sit on him and watch him as we fucked. I placed his long, hard cock deep inside me. The feeling was so intense. I felt him pushing against my G-spot as our bodies began to sweat. I pushed my breasts up against his chest and kissed him deeply. My legs wrapped around the seat, I pulled his ass closer to me as I rocked him hard. I could feel my ass bouncing against his legs. Both of his hands reached up to couple my breasts as he held them and pinched at my nipples.

I was sucking his neck, licking his eyelids, my hands holding his hair. I pushed his face into my chest, his mouth on my nipples as I squeezed him tighter and tighter until I was going to explode. As if he read my mind, he gave one long thrust and I felt hot liquid inside me.

Shaking, I came with him, the intensity wracking my body, sweat dripping down his chest, the cool night air blowing my hair. We stayed like that for a while, each of them revelling in the beauty of the act.

I kissed him long, and hard and felt him growing hard again inside me. Slowly I removed him. He slid out from under my body and opened the car door. Placing me on my stomach, he demanded that I grab hold of the stick shift. Standing behind me, he took my legs and wrapped them around his waist. He wanted me again, this time from behind. He stood between my legs and pushed his hardened dick deep inside me. He slammed me again and again and with each thrust smiled at the deepness

216 **SEX FANTASIES BY WOMEN FOR WOMEN**

of the penetration. I moved in the same rhythm with him, saying nothing, but rocking and moving just the same.

This time he couldn't hold his orgasm, as he gave me a final push, both hands on my ass, he grabbed me by the waist to reach up to him. His release was solid and he filled me with his hot cum. I arched my back, grabbing the stick, feeling the warmth and my orgasm as well, I pushed into him fully, until I could hold him no more. He withdrew and with one hand against the small of my back, traced the wetness of my sweat. I lay there breathing quietly for a bit, as he began to dress.

He handed me a towel that he had stashed in the back and when I went to clean myself, took the towel away and wiped myself tenderly. Kneeling in front of me, he helped me to put the dress back over my head. He cupped my face and kissed me lightly.

He walked to the driver's side and stepped in. Starting the car, he gently backed onto the highway. The only thing remaining, was the light of the full right moon. Both of us smiling, we made our way back home.

Carla, 29, executive

This is a letter I received from an old boyfriend. He said he had been fantasizing about me and felt he had to share what he had been thinking with me. The letter threw me, because frankly, during sex, he had never been very giving and this was one of the reasons we broke up. Since receiving the letter, we have spoken on the phone several times and are thinking about getting back together. Here is the letter:

'You are lying on your stomach on the bed. You have no clothes on. The light from the scented candles reflects off the oil I am massaging into your skin. John Coltrane is playing softly on the stereo as I slowly work the tension out of your upper back.

'I'm moving down your back rubbing with a circular motion, taking my time (what's the hurry?) and the tension that has built up during the long work week is melting away.

'I work my way down your lower back, your buttocks, your thighs, your calves and now I'm massaging your feet.

'I ask you to turn over and you do. I am overwhelmed, once again, by the sight of your body. Your nipples are pointing straight up in the air and your pussy is wet and swollen. I can smell you and I have to resist the urge to just plunge inside you at this moment.

'I begin my work again this time starting at your temples. You are surprised at the tension there and become even more aroused as the muscles in your face relax. I'm working my way down now, massaging your cheeks, your neck, your shoulders.

'After I have massaged your arms I am working under your arms and the sides of your breasts, carefully avoiding your nipples which seem to have grown even more erect. Now across your stomach and down to your hips. As I ease down to your thighs, avoiding your bush, you let out a small whimper and thrust your mound up at me.

'But it's not quite time for that. After I've worked my way back down to your feet and massaged your toes you are lying almost asleep. Your eyes are closed but the scent of your arousal gives you away. You are not asleep. You are waiting.

'Now your eyes are still closed and you feel the gentlest of kisses on your lips. You open your mouth and I gently suck the tip of your tongue into mine. I leave your mouth and begin to nibble on your neck while I knead your breasts with a lust that I cannot hold back any longer. I suck one nipple and then the other as my hand moves down to your dripping cunt. I cup your pussy in my right hand and you lift your hips off the bed to push against it.

'I pull back now and look at you. You're breathing hard, your nipples are erect and your pussy is sopping wet. You look up at me confused, as if to say, "Why are you stopping? Don't stop."

'Now you're ready.

'I tell you to turn over on your stomach and tuck your knees up to your chest. You still seem confused but you do as your told. I kneel behind you and begin to rub your pussy. You're surprised when you feel my tongue begin to probe your asshole but you relax when you realize how good it feels. I'm pumping three fingers in and out of your cunt-hole hard and fast and now I pull all the way out and plunge back in with four. My tongue is as far up your back door as it can go and now as I fuck you with four fingers I begin to rub your clit with my thumb. That's what sends you over the edge.

'You're screaming now and pumping your ass in the air in rhythm to my fingers. You're coming but at the same time there's an unfamiliar feeling in your ass. You've never felt this way before and you're not quite sure what to do about it but suddenly my tongue is not enough. You feel a void that needs to be filled. It hits you like a punch to the stomach; you need my cock up your ass. You crave it and now you have to have it. You beg me, plead with me. You need it and you need it right now. I'm happy to oblige. I reach over and get some KY jelly.

'I lube up my prick quickly and position it at your entrance. You feel my stiff cock poised to enter you and slam yourself back onto it. It pops right in and I can't believe how good it feels inside your tight ass. You pause a second and then pull forward until just the head of my cock is still inside you then you slam back against me again. I'm pumping your ass good now while you furiously rub your clit. You're close now, I can feel it.

'I am getting ready now and I tell you so. You tell me to come. You want to feel it shoot up your ass and you begin to pump against me even more violently (we're both going to be sore and bruised in the morning.) I feel my balls begin to tighten up and now I'm coming. I'm up inside your ass as far as I can go pumping wave after wave of hot come into you. I feel your whole body begin to shake as your final orgasm hits you. With my cock inside you I can feel every muscle in your ass and cunt spasm.

'You're lying on your side now with me right behind you. My cock is still firmly planted in your ass and I can feel an occasional aftershock spasm run through you. In a little while my dick will shrink and plop out of you and my come will be oozing out. For now though you're lying in my arms as we listen to the sweet music and bask in the afterglow.'

Marybeth, 28, photographer

I got home from work one Friday, feeling somewhat kinky and in the mood for something wild and crazy. I went to the bedroom and stripped out of my work clothes, then to the bathroom for a relaxing bath. I began to wash myself, sliding my soapy hand over my neck to my breasts, down my stomach then down between my legs, and began playing with myself thinking about having sex with my husband and another man at the same time.

I imagined my husband watching and that made it even sexier. I began whispering to myself over and over, 'Fuck me, fuck me,' almost feeling the warmth of his own climax enter my body, filling every inch inside of me. Then I came. I laid in the hot tub for several minutes as the vision faded along with my orgasm.

I have shared this fantasy with my husband and he thinks it is really sexy.

Marla, 22, nanny

I read this story in a book once. Since, I've put myself in the starring role.

I arrive at the hotel, already dressed in my little schoolgirl outfit. I get some curious looks from people in the lobby, but I really don't care. After ducking into the restroom briefly to fix up my hair, I quickly make my way to Room 107. I knock on the door, and a man is quick to answer it.

'Hi, I'm Marla,' I say shyly, and he opens the door with a smile.

'Hi, I. Wow! I'm John ... Come on in!'

I walk into the room as John closes the door and bolts it.

'Hey, Mike!' he calls into the bathroom. 'You've got to see this girl!' I blush as Mike walks into the room.

'Holy shit ...' Mike mutters. The two men gawk over sweet young I, dressed in my little schoolgirl outfit.

I am wearing a crisp, long-sleeved white blouse, with a red/black/yellow plaid necktie. My torso is caressed by a matching buttoned-down red/black/yellow plaid vest, which fits snugly, accentuating my firm teenaged breasts and flat tummy. My skirt is made from the same plaid fabric, layered in tiny knife-pleats, riding high on my lovely thin thighs. My white cable-knit knee socks and black-and-white saddle shoes complete my sweet outfit nicely. My lips shine with my red lipstick, and my hair is swept to the sides in two ponytails, with bangs draping across my forehead.

I am enjoying playing the part of an innocent little girl, and I sway from side to side slightly, like a nervous youngster.

'Do you like my outfit?' I ask, spinning around for the guys. My flimsy, lightweight skirt flares out its pleats and gives the horny men a fleeting glimpse of sweet white cotton panties.

'Shit, yes!' John blurts.

'What did you guys want me for, anyway?' I ask, teasingly.

Mike smiles at me, stepping up to me. He patts my ass lightly through my little pleated skirt. 'It all depends,' answers Mike. 'Are you a good little girl, or a naughty girl?'

'Well, most of the time, I'm good, but when I'm naughty, I'm even better ...' I reply, with the wink of an eye.

'Well, now, my little sweetheart,' Mike answers, 'let's see just what a naughty little schoolgirl you are ...'

The radio in the room is playing a very sensuous song, and I decide to use it to enhance my teen charms. I sit in a chair across from the bed. The men sit on the bed, watching me intently. I put a saddle shoe up on an armrest, and cock the other leg wide to the other side. My little school skirt drapes down across the gap between my legs.

Mike and John are mesmerized. I am simply delightful in my little uniform. As they watch, I slowly slide my plaid pleated skirt up over my tight white panties, showing them my lovely panty-covered crotch. I am loving every minute of this.

SEX FANTASIES BY WOMEN FOR WOMEN

I slowly slide a finger in through the leg-band of my panties, probing my wetness, moaning softly to add to the effect. I can see their jeans begin to bulge ominously.

I continue to finger myself, my fingers moving in and out of my teen cunt under the panties, my knuckles stretching out the fabric. My other hand slowly unbuttons my vest and begins massaging my breasts through my soft white blouse. 'Would you guys like to see my little pussy?' I ask.

'Oh, yeah ...' they both mutter, horny as hell.

I hook a finger around a leg-band and pull the fabric to the side, exposing my treasure. The soft curls of pussy hair are glistening with my moisture, and the sight of it, coupled with the school uniform and my provocative pose, is enough to almost make the guys come in their pants right then and there.

'God, I could cum right now!' gasps John.

'Oh, no, don't do that right now,' I say. 'You've got to fuck me, first! Let's see those cocks ...'

The men quickly strip before me. In seconds, their clothes are thrown aside, with both men standing before me, their pricks hard and lewdly wobbling in worship to my charms. The men pull me up from the chair and bring me to the bed.

'Hey, John, why don't you let her suck you while I eat her pussy?' Mike suggest.

'Great idea!' John quickly agrees. He stretches out on the bed, his head propped up on a pillow. Mike reaches up under my flimsy little skirt and thumbs my panties down, tugging them over my precious ass cheeks, till they fall to the floor. I toss my vest to the floor. I crawl onto the bed, slowly moving my way up between John's legs to his waiting 7-inch schlong.

As I grip John's warm, hard cock in one hand, I can feel my little skirt pulled up high on the back of my ass, high in the air as I kneel on the bed, and the wonderful sensation of a man's tongue on my pussy lips.

I know I am going to really enjoy this night.

I have shared parts of it with my boyfriend – like being ravished by two men at the same time, but his reaction has made me think he would get upset if he knew just how detailed the fantasy is and how often I think of it when we make love. He was intrigued but also slightly put out, like he thought HE should be enough for me and I shouldn't be fantasizing about anything else. He is, but I think that fantasy is a huge part of what makes sex sexy. I wish he could understand that.

Adrienne, 18, hostess

My boyfriend recently told me that he loves girls wearing their hair in two braided pigtails, that it looks innocent and sweet and sexy at the same time to him. He says he thinks teenage girls are really sexy to look at though he wouldn't want to actually be with one as he thinks they're really shallow and inexperienced. Recently I have got this fantasy on my mind: I buy some teenage girl style (bright colours and tight clothing) and put them on and we fuck our brains out. I shared my idea with him and he is really into it.

Deborah, 29, accountant

One fall weekend, my husband and I rented a condo on the beach. We found all these pornographic magazines with unbelievably explicit stories left by the previous occupants. Women screwing dogs, other women, 16 men. Even though they turned me on and I know they had the same effect on my husband (I could see him hardening), we were too embarrassed to admit it. Instead, we laughed and threw them out. But now I imagine what would have happened if we had been braver and read them to each other by the fire as the sun went down over the water. We would have made sweet beautiful love all weekend and maybe tried some new things (do I need to say that our sex life is a bit stale?).

Sometimes I fantasize that I have found the magazines and somehow they become real. As I am being screwed by a dog and another woman, my husband walks in. He says he didn't know I was so sexy and starts to make love to me. The dog and the woman disappear and it's just us.

I tried telling my husband about my fantasy but I could tell that he didn't want to hear. Although he satisfies me, our sex is a bit boring. He can be quite close-mouthed about what turns him on – which is probably why we didn't do anything more than flip through the magazines in the first place. There are a lot of things I know make him horny – like the thought of two women making love (he practically had a hard-on throughout the entire movie *Bound*), but he would never admit it. It makes me sort of sad because I think our love life could be much more exciting than it is.

living
them out

Introduction

(Some) fantasies are worth living out. If you're in a long-term relationship that's lost a little of its sizzle, or if you're in a new relationship with someone and you discover you've always had the same secret desire, then you might want to figure out how to make one or more of your wilder fantasies come true.

Some, of course, can never be lived out, especially those that go against the laws of physics, the laws of nature or the laws of your local police. But as long as you have another consenting adult willing to play your fantasies out, then with a little effort and a little imagination, you can make a sexual adventure you'll never forget.

That's not to say that you should rush in and tell your partner how much you'd like to find his best friend's marvellously buffed pecs underneath the tree this Christmas. Start with fantasies that involve your lover, ones that he might enjoy playing out, too. This way you'll be helping to increase the intimacy in your relationship.

Also, be aware that a fantasy is always in your control. Real life is very different: You're negotiating with a partner; it may be cloudy outside, it may not be as enticing as you had imagined watching your lover caress someone else. Which is why many of the responses we had on making sexual fantasies a reality were mixed – for some, it was an incredible turn-on; for others, an event that soured their relationship. There's no way to predict which way it will go – which may be why we received the fewest responses in this category – most people realize that their fantasies are just that – and have no desire to make them the real thing. The experts agree – most advise that the best place for acting out your fantasy is your imagination.

Kellie, 28, writer

I actually WAS in a threesome once, with my boyfriend and a male friend of ours – it was his birthday present.

However, there was no touching between the two guys, except maybe the heads of their cocks touching in my mouth when I sucked them both off at the same time.

My boyfriend loved it and I liked being with two guys at the same time. But I am somewhat bi-curious, and would love to explore being with another girl as well. The thought of licking a woman's clit while a man is fucking her really turns me on, and I'd like to take it out of her pussy, give it a good suck, and then place it back inside her. I think my boyfriend would be into it.

The best would be two couples – and anything goes ...

My boyfriend and I are really open with each other sexually – more so than I have been with any other guy and I have had the best sex that I have ever had with him.

Terri, 29, chemist

I recently met my online lover for our first 'real' encounter, although we both felt like we knew each other very well for several months prior to meeting in person. Anyone who has experienced the joy of an intimate cyber relationship knows what I'm talking about.

We live several hundred miles apart so I flew to his city for our day together. During the two hour flight, a million thoughts ran through my head, all of them positive. I knew in my heart this man and I would connect in all the sensual and loving ways we had in cyberspace. My conversation with fellow passengers sitting near me was lively and enthusiastic. I couldn't help but let the building excitement and anticipation shine through in my outward attitude. Anyone could see and hear my obvious happiness.

When the plane landed and I walked into the terminal, he was right there waiting for me with the look of love in his eyes. I will never forget that expression and how I felt when I first saw him. It is etched in my mind forever. We were instantly at ease with each other, no awkward moments interfering in any way with our pleasure. Together we walked hand in hand to his car, but once in the parking garage we could no longer resist the temptation to experience our first kiss ... in person. We had made love to each other online so many, many times prior to that day. When our lips met in 'reality', our bodies finally became one just as our hearts and minds had already done in the weeks and months leading to that moment. We looked into each other's eyes and smiled, knowing the magic we felt in our cyber home would indeed be with us in the hotel room that waited.

It was. We spent the next eight hours locked away from the world around us as if we truly were the only two people on the face of this earth. We went to paradise and back together several times that day. It was by far the most erotic and completely satisfying experience I have ever had. It was also the most meaningful, and unfortunately bittersweet. He and I are both married to others. We knew from the beginning of our relationship that there were great obstacles and risks to complicate what we felt for each other, and make being together difficult and at times truly impossible. Ignoring all else, we followed our passion and love. We're both grateful for and in awe of the experience, and do plan to repeat it again when we can. We love and desire each other and have grown to accept being together emotionally even though we are physically apart. It isn't always easy and it does cause frustration and pain. But anything worth having is a struggle at times. We face the challenge together and do so with understanding, consideration, and endless love.

I'm sharing this as an example that cyber love can be as fulfilling as any other kind ... in many ways even more so, at least for me. This man brings me more joy than I could ever express with words. We have no desire or intention of hurting the others we love in this world. Our only reason for being together is to enhance each other's daily lives with the love and incredible sensuality we give and take in our relationship. It makes us both happier, kinder people to everyone around us.

Rowena, 31, insurance

After reading your request for fantasies, I just have to tell you what happened to me a couple of nights ago.

I was out of town on a business trip, and spent three nights in a motel. On the second night, I had finished work, had a shower, changed into casual clothes and went to the dining room for a meal. I sat at the bar for a drink while looking at the menu, and a few minutes after I sat down, another woman on her own came in and sat at the other end of the bar. I felt her eyes watching me, and after a few minutes, made eye contact with her and smiled. Thinking nothing more of it, I ordered my meal and went to a table to eat.

Her eyes kept on watching me. Then she came over and said that she hated eating by herself and would I mind if she joined me at my table. I figured that she might be interesting company, so I agreed. She said her name was Melanie, and was a sales rep for a shoe company. She ordered a bottle of white wine for us to share, and we chatted casually as we ate and enjoyed the wine.

As dinner progressed, she became more friendly towards me. Her smile was amazing, and I was beginning to find her hazel eyes quite captivating. Melanie was flirting with me! Her head was at that angle; her smile had that look, and I was beginning to enjoy it. I was feeling quite flattered, and wondered where it was going. I didn't have to wait long to find out!

As we finished the main course, Melanie asked me if I was married. She was, and her husband also travelled with his work and they only met at weekends. She said she got very horny in between times, finding time alone in a motel room very boring. I told her I was single, but had a regular guy who I saw most weekends. Did I get horny while travelling, she asked. Well, I had to reply 'yes' and then out it came. Did I feel horny enough to do it with her tonight?

My pussy was getting wet, but all my senses were confused. Should I or shouldn't I? Melanie didn't live in my town and I thought the chances of ever seeing her again were slim, so if it was a disaster I wouldn't ever have to face her again. I'd been with a couple of girls before; a couple of three-ways and the other was a school friend who I had known for ages and been with a few times. But Melanie was a total stranger. I said yes.

We went to her room and what happened for the next few hours was just bliss. Never did I imagine that it could be this good. Melanie slowly undressed me, licking and kissing every inch of me. When I was totally naked, she lay me on the bed and stripped off in front of me. I couldn't help myself. My fingers were working my pussy, deeper, harder, until I came watching her. It took her at least 10 minutes to undress, caressing her tits, thighs and pussy until she lowered herself to my gushing hole. She drank from me. Tongue deep inside me until I felt I would burst. Then she slowly pushed her fingers and then her hand into me until her fist was buried inside me.

Her kiss on my lips was electric. Her hand inside me was wonderful. No guy had ever been able to do that to me but because Melanie had taken so much time, and I was so ready, it was easy. My second orgasm was the strongest I'd ever experienced.

Now she said, it's your turn. Her fist came out, and she pushed me down to her slit. Smooth, deep red and so wet. My fingers explored her clit, swollen and firm. I teased her by feather touching her cunt, and she was thrusting herself upwards to meet my touch. Finally I went in. Harder she moaned, harder. Both hands were working her, along with my tongue. I moved one finger to her bum and entered it; my other hand in her pussy. I licked her clit – it tasted so good. Then she came. Gushed more like. Oceans of it everywhere. She collapsed and we melted into the longest, tastiest kiss I could imagine. It lasted for ages, and we topped up each other's taste buds with our pussy juices.

Melanie got up and brought a banana back to bed. Unpeeling it, she slowly inserted one end into her and got me to put the other end into me. Closer and closer until we were rubbing pussy to pussy. Her fingers on my clit, mine on hers. After we both came again, I ate her end of the banana and she ate the end that had been in me. We kissed again and fell asleep.

I woke at 3am and we fingered each other to orgasm again and tit-fucked each other. I dressed and went back to my room and when I got up at 7, her car was gone.

God, I miss her.

Sara, 23, nanny

My fantasies change because they depend on people I meet and fancy. Mark, an ex of mine, had a really gorgeous friend called Christopher. He had curly blonde hair and looked like a rock star. He was also totally unattainable to me because he wouldn't date a friend's ex. We'd often crash at his flat and I would masturbate (after making sure Mark was asleep) then Christopher would slip into bed with us, desperate to have me. We'd start teasing at each other and then he'd drag me off to his bedroom to have sex. It was great until Mark caught us – which is why we broke up!

Marcia, 26, customer services operator

While on holiday this year, my boyfriend was feeling horny so we started having sex. I've always been turned on at the thought of being watched and so has he. Bearing this in mind, he started fucking me up against a wall which looked directly out of some patio doors to the road below. While we were going at it, I said if anyone looks up they will be able to see us. As soon as I said this, he moved round so he was in the doorway fucking me from behind. A couple walking by saw us and gave us a smile and a wave, which certainly turned us on. I lost count of the number of times I came and when my boyfriend shot his load, it was like never before. I guess we both like being watched and watching for that matter.

Andrea, 28, credit controller

I like the idea of being watched and regularly fantasize about masturbating in front of my bedroom window and being seen. A really good-looking guy moved into an apartment slightly above me. I can see straight into his bedroom and would regularly masturbate in the shadows while watching him get dressed and undressed. One day, I decided to make my fantasy come true and so got naked and left on my lights. When he came in, I made a few movements to catch his eye and then cautiously turned and revealed myself.

Immediate reaction? An almost derisive snort, laugh, or something like that, so I covered up immediately.

When he looked again, however, I showed myself, this time boldly, and began masturbating. This was the beginning of a long 'relationship', a pleasure indulged in at least once a day, whenever his wife and my husband were both away for at least a few hot minutes.

Jan, 26, accountant

My boyfriend and I pretend I am an expensive call girl. Men make appointments weeks in advance to have sex with me. My boyfriend is one of my clients and I give him the best time he's ever had in bed. I know he'll be back again and again.

We tried acting out another fantasy of mine where he 'rapes' me, but that wasn't as exciting as I had imagined, so we didn't do it again.

Anonymous

I often had fantasies about a black man making love to me. He has a large penis and stays erect a long, long time. Then I seduced a black man at my gym. Boy, what a surprise! He was puny and really nervous and inept. I ended up jacking myself off and thinking about my fantasy in order to come!

Susan, 29, nurse

I have had lots of fantasies. A lot I try to live out. But when I do, I have noticed I don't have the fantasy as much any more. For instance, making love on a remote beach. I used to have that all the time, but my lover and I did it when we were on holiday in Turkey last year and now I don't have it as much any more. Same goes for making love in a threesome. I did that with a close girlfriend and her boyfriend and it wasn't how I had fantasized it at all – too many people to take care of at once! A current fantasy is to make love outside under a sky full of stars. Hopefully, I'll do this soon too.

Anna, 28, data programmer

My fave fantasy is actually one that I have lived out. I'd always had the fantasy of sleeping with another woman and the fantasy came true when I found a boyfriend as liberal-minded as myself.

We went along to a party that catered especially for people who are sexually liberated. We were surprised and nervous when we first arrived, the surroundings were relaxing. The room was decorated in deep red and purple colours with velvet cushions, everything felt very luxurious. We had a few drinks and got chatting to the female host of the party. She was very friendly and helped us to relax a lot more.

As the evening progressed, the hostess flirted with both of us so we progressed upstairs into a room that was also decorated in red and purple with a large mattress on the floor. My boyfriend and I started to kiss and the hostess began to run her fingers across my back.

It was electric, just that slight touch, in the anticipation of what was about to happen. I turned to softly kiss the hostess. It wasn't like a man's kiss – it was gentler and slower. I began to caress her breasts, removing her clothes, feeling the softness of her skin.

She threw me over onto the mattress and started to trace her tongue slowly down my body, I knew what was about to happen and I couldn't wait. She started to go down on me whilst my boyfriend kissed me and caressed my breasts. The evening progressed into the early hours of the morning. I can't remember everything that happened but it included my boyfriend and I making love with the hostess.

Strangely enough, the evening brought us both closer because now we both have a secret that nobody else outside of that party would ever knows about. We have many more fantasies that we hope to live out together.

Megan, 29, laboratory technician

Living with Mitch for three years means that our sex life has become pretty routine. We still have good sex, but it's not hot passion any more. Then a friend confided she and her boyfriend had had a foursome. By the time she filled me in on the juicy details, I was really turned on. That night, when I made love to Mitch, I was rampant. He asked what had gotten into me. I was embarrassed but told him about my friend and the foursome. Mitch admitted he'd always fantasized about having sex with two women.

For the next few weeks, our sex life was really exciting. We fantasized about having a threesome and touched each other in ways that made it feel like here was another person in bed with us. But we never talked about doing it for real.

Then one night I went out clubbing with my girlfriend. We came back to my place at 3am, completely drunk. Mitch was still up watching TV. We stayed up chatting and the conversation strayed to sex.

Mitch asked Tammy if she'd ever fantasized about sleeping with another woman. She smiled and said all women did. We talked some more then Mitch said he was turning in. I started to follow him when he turned to Tammy and asked her if she wanted to join us. I was shocked when she said yes.

We went into the bedroom, stripped off and got into bed, Tammy was in the middle. At first, we were all shy and giggling, but Mitch took the lead and started to touch Tammy.

That's when the jealousy started – Mitch was MY boyfriend. Surely WE should have started things off. Feeling like a gooseberry, I stroked Tammy's back while he kissed and fondled her. After a while, I started to get turned on. I wanted to join in so I eased Tammy across to me and kissed her on the lips. I'd never kissed a woman before, but it was such a turn-on I forgot about Mitch.

Mitch watched as Tammy and I masturbated each other. The he pulled Tammy across to him and began to make love to her. He wasn't interested in me at all. I felt hurt.

In my fantasies, we all touched each other at once, that wasn't how things were going. I felt like I was there just to give Mitch permission to have sex with Tammy. The booze was wearing off, the fantasy was becoming real and it was out of control. The idea of a threesome was great but my boyfriend was having sex with my best friend and I didn't like it. I pulled Mitch off Tammy and said I wanted it to stop. They were confused and Tammy left, crying. In the morning I was still angry and upset. Mitch couldn't understand it. I think men are better at separating sex and love. We broke up a week later and Tammy and I haven't spoken since.

Karen, 22, student

I had this fantasy about making love quietly among a group of people. I was at a party where everyone was crashing around us and my boyfriend and I were a bit drunk and horny so I whispered it to him. Later, when we were half-asleep, lying on the floor next to a few friends, he started rubbing his body against mine. Then he eased himself inside me and we had sex. There were lots of sleeping bodies around us, but we were totally oblivious to them. It's exactly how I'd fantasized it – that dozy, cosy kind of sex when you're half-asleep and your mind and body are really relaxed.

Gina, 30, insurance underwriter

I had this fantasy about a young boy that I tried making real. The boy was doing some lawn work for me. He was young and shy. In my fantasy, I spend the afternoon with him and slowly seduce him, caressing him and tongue-licking his body as I undress him. He loses his inhibitions and we make sweet love. But in reality, he came as soon as I kissed him and was so embarrassed that he started crying!

Barbara, 27, supervisor

I always fantasize about making it with another woman and a guy. I recently had the chance to do it – it was soooo incredibly sexy! The first time it happened like this: I was skinny dipping with my friend Ben (as we did a lot in the summers together) and as we were sunning dry he said, 'You have a great body. I've been thinking about this for a while – would you like to have a threesome with Susan and me? I've asked her and she said she'd love it.' I agreed.

She welcomed us into her bedroom and told us both to take off our clothes, sit in some chairs at the foot of the bed and watch her. She took off her robe, sat on the bed facing us with her legs spread wide and proceeded to stroke her beautiful, pink pussy until she was totally soaking wet and purring BIG time. I was dripping wet and Ben was rock hard by the time she was done.

Susan told us, 'Okay, you're ready now.' She turned to me. 'Barbara, open me up so I can take all of Ben's length. I don't think I'll be able to without you opening me up good.' She asked me to finger her from behind and she bit her lower lip hard as I drove my fingers deeper and deeper and deeper into her lovely tight wet pussy. Soon she took as much of Ben's cock into her mouth as she could possibly take. As I finger-fucked her as deep as I could reach, my head was beside hers and I could see everything she was doing to my friend's cock up close. Incredibly delicious!!!

After a while, she told Ben, 'I'm ready to take you into me now.' We switched places and as she kissed and sucked her juices off my fingers and fingered me, I watched her take ALL of his cock into her. With the last inch fully inside her, she came so hard she cried – tears streamed down her face as she begged me to play with her clit. I came as she was still coming. 'OMIGOD FUCK ME as hard and as deep as you can ... That's it ... oh lover, that's it ... fuck me ... fuck me ...' She licked her juices off Ben's cock as I finger-fucked her HARD again and she came again and again. We switched back and forth over and over until finally she said she couldn't take any more.

101 NIGHTS OF TANTRIC SEX
How to Make Each Night a New Way to Sexual Ecstasy

Cassandra Lorius

Switch off the mind, awaken all the senses and become aware of your whole body with this superbly illustrated guide to using and enhancing Tantric sexual energy.

Tantra, the Tao of Love, is an Eastern path to self-development. Central to that path is healthy sexual energy, which needs to be harmonized if we're to live life happily and fulfil our true potential. The Tantra involves letting your mind go and learning to express yourself through your body, nurturing intimacy, sexual and emotional self-confidence and the healthy development of sexual energy flow through the whole body.

101 Nights of Tantric Sex leads you through 101 nights of rituals and meditations to bring you closer to the divine, including:

- Affirming your commitment
- Playing the Yin-Yang game
- Honouring your partner
- Creating sacred space
- Erotic touch
- Co-mingling breath
- Anointing the Chakras

ISBN 0 00 713273 5

Order a copy now at www.thorsons.com

THE ULTIMATE KAMA SUTRA IN A BOX

Learn the sensuous and erotic art of lovemaking from the Kama Sutra, the all-time classic and the most famous book on the art and skills of sex and love ever written, in this beautifully illustrated and easy-to-use introductory guide, which includes a 96-page book as well as 30 full-colour 'how-to' cards.

The Kama Sutra teaches that lovemaking should be an ecstatic experience, but sexual happiness can only occur if both partners have a good understanding of the practical side of sex as well as the emotional issues that surround it. Following the original texts of the most famous book ever written on the art and skills of sex and love, *The Ultimate Kama Sutra in a Box* presents sensuous techniques, sexual positions and creative ideas for enriched lovemaking in an innovative and easy-to-follow format.

Embracing the spiritual side of love and sex, the illustrated introductory book and 30 full-colour step-by-step cards open up a realm of new and erotic possibilities that will create profound changes in your sex life. This is the ultimate guide for lovers, presented in a new and original way.

ISBN 0 00 714753 8

Order a copy now at www.thorsons.com